PLANT-BASED
DIET
COOKBOOK
FOR BEGINNERS

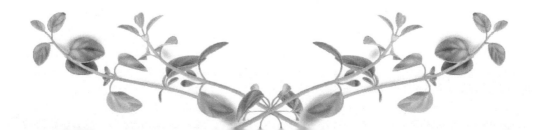

DISCLAIMER

The information provided in this book is for educational and informational purposes only and should not be construed as medical or health advice. This book contains the author's opinions and does not intend to replace professional medical advice, diagnosis, or treatment. Readers should always consult their healthcare provider before making health-related decisions or for counseling, guidance, and treatment about a specific medical condition.

Melody Reeves, while not a physician, provides advice based on her own experiences and extensive research. The dietary practices described in the book are based on thorough research and personal experiences, but individual results may vary. Readers should use their discretion and consider their health conditions (or consult a healthcare professional) before adopting any nutritional or lifestyle changes.

The author and publisher disclaim any liability directly or indirectly for anyone using this book's material.

Table of Contents

Introduction

Welcome to the beginning of your vibrant culinary journey—where freshness meets flavor, and every meal nourishes your body and soul. Whether taking your first steps toward a plant-based diet for health reasons, ethical concerns, environmental considerations, or perhaps a combination of all three, you've made a transformative choice.

Imagine walking into your kitchen, feeling confident and excited to prepare meals as nutritious as they are delicious. Picture the vibrant colors of fresh produce on your countertop, the rich aromas filling your kitchen, and the joy of knowing that your cooking is pleasing your palate and protecting the planet. This isn't just an aspiration—it's your new reality as you flip through the pages of this book.

You may wonder, "Can I make tasty meals out of plants?" or "Isn't a plant-based diet limiting?" Let me assure you that as you delve into the chapters of this book, you will discover the joy and creativity of plant-based cooking. Each recipe is designed not only to guide you but also to inspire your culinary creativity. The beauty of these recipes lies in their flexibility—feel free to substitute ingredients based on availability or your preference. No cilantro? Use parsley! No apple? How about a pear? This book encourages you to use what you have, reducing waste and stress. Here, cooking becomes an act of joy and inspiration rather than just a necessity.

Embarking on this plant-based eating path might seem daunting at first. You might worry about missing your favorite dishes or needing more protein. These are typical concerns for anyone adopting a new way of eating. However, within these pages lies a treasure trove of recipes that reimagine classic favorites and introduce you to new staples. You'll learn how to cook hearty, satisfying meals that nourish you and are light and delightful.

The transformation goes beyond your plate. Adopting a plant-based diet can lead to profound changes in your health—imagine fewer digestive issues, reduced risk of chronic diseases, and a feeling of general well-being. You may benefit from increased energy and positive changes in your skin and hair. The plant-based lifestyle is a powerful way to align your health goals with your values, leading to a fulfilling and sustainable way of living. Rest assured, your health is in good hands with a plant-based diet.

So, turn the page and begin the delicious, healthful, and ethically rewarding journey together.

Chapter 1:

THE FUNDAMENTALS OF PLANT-BASED DIET

Switching to Plant-Based - The Seamless Transition

Embarking on a plant-based journey doesn't have to be a radical overnight change. Instead, view it as continuous improvement to your diet, each step adding more health and vitality to your life. This chapter will break down the transition into simple, doable steps to make the shift enjoyable, empowering and delicious.

Start Small: Begin by integrating plant-based meals into your diet one day at a time. Designate one day a week as a plant-based day. Popular initiatives like "Meatless Monday" can provide structure and a support community to make this transition smoother. This isn't just about subtracting from your diet; it's about adding diversity, colors, and flavors.

Educate Yourself: Knowledge is power. Understand the nutritional bases of your meals and what your body needs. This ensures that you're not just eating plant-based, but you're eating well. Familiarize yourself with plant protein sources, the importance of whole grains, and where to find essential fats. Books, documentaries, and even plant-based cooking classes can be invaluable resources.

Revamp Your Pantry: Gradually replace processed foods with whole-food alternatives. Stock up on legumes, whole grains, nuts, seeds, and spices. A well-stocked pantry is your best defense against the temptation to discard less healthy options. It also makes preparing delicious plant-based meals a straightforward and spontaneous part of your daily life.

Experiment with Recipes: Let your kitchen be your laboratory. Experimenting with recipes is fun and allows you to discover new favorite dishes that can replace old, less healthy cravings. Online platforms and cookbooks are gold mines for tried-and-tested recipes that can guide you in expanding your culinary repertoire.

Connect with a Community: You're not alone in this journey. Connecting with others transitioning to a plant-based diet can provide motivation, inspiration, and practical tips. Community connections can be incredibly supportive, Whether through online forums, local groups, or potluck dinners.

Be Patient and Persistent: Change takes time. Your taste buds and cooking skills will evolve. What seems unfamiliar now will soon become second nature. Celebrate small victories along the way, and don't be too hard on yourself during setbacks. Consistency is vital, not perfection.

By taking these steps, shifting to a plant-based lifestyle can be a smooth and enjoyable adventure. Remember, this is about creating a sustainable, healthful way of eating that energizes and rejuvenates your body. Welcome to a vibrant new way of living where your diet is not just about nourishment but also pleasure and discovery.

The Metabolic Plate Method: Simplifying Nutritional Basics

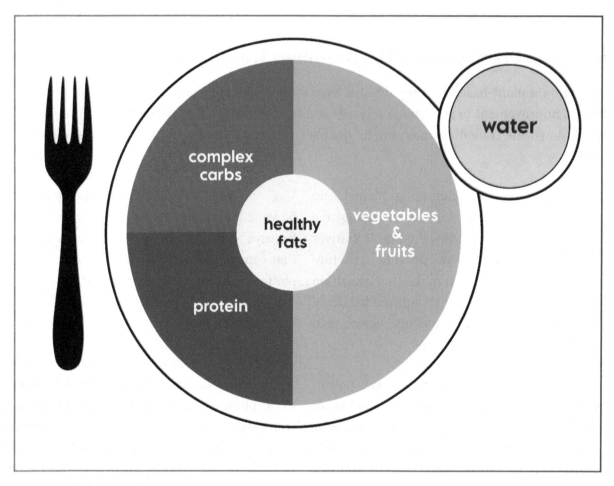

Maintaining a balanced diet can seem like a complex puzzle in today's fast-paced world. The Metabolic Plate Method offers a straightforward solution that simplifies nutritional balance by visually dividing your plate to ensure a healthy, well-rounded meal without the need for calorie counting or nutrient tracking.

Essentials of the Metabolic Plate Method

This approach simplifies meal planning by dividing the plate into three key sections:

- **Proteins (25% of the plate):** Include high-quality protein sources, which are essential for building and repairing tissues and supporting immune function. Plant-based options like legumes, tofu, and tempeh provide protein and other health benefits such as fiber and reduced saturated fat intake.

- **Vegetables and Fruits (50% of the plate):** Occupying half of the plate, this section is dedicated to vegetables and fruits, which are rich in vitamins, minerals, fiber, and antioxidants. These components are essential for reducing the risk of chronic diseases and maintaining overall health. The variety in colors and types ensures a broad variety of nutrients.

- **Carbohydrates (25% of the plate):** The remaining quarter should be filled with whole grains like brown rice, whole wheat, quinoa, or starchy vegetables such as sweet potatoes. These carbohydrates are vital for providing energy, improving digestion, and helping regulate blood sugar levels.

Alignment with Harvard's Healthy Eating Plate

The Metabolic Plate Method mirrors the guidelines recommended by Harvard's Healthy Eating Plate, emphasizing the importance of the quality and proportion of the foods consumed. According to Harvard, a balanced plate helps tackle dietary deficiencies and excesses without complex calculations, focusing instead on dietary quality and variety.

Life Simplified

Adopting the Metabolic Plate Method simplifies eating healthily by:

- **Eliminating the Need for Calorie Counting:** By following this visual guide, you can easily maintain a balanced intake of proteins, carbohydrates, and fats without having to measure or calculate calories.

- **Ensuring Nutritional Completeness:** This method encourages a varied diet that includes all the essential nutrients required for good health, and reduces the risk of nutrient deficiencies.

- **Promoting Satiety and Reducing Cravings:** The high fiber content from fruits and vegetables, combined with protein and good fats, fosters a feeling of fullness and helps curb cravings for unhealthy snacks and sugary foods.

Application Across All Meals

Whether it's breakfast, lunch, or dinner, the Metabolic Plate Method provides a consistent framework for healthy eating. Here are some examples:

- **Breakfast:** Your plate might include scrambled tofu (protein), a side of mixed berries and spinach (vegetables and fruits), and a slice of whole-grain toast (carbohydrates).

- **Lunch:** A salad with chickpeas or lentils (protein), a variety of leafy greens and colorful vegetables (vegetables and fruits), and a quinoa salad (carbohydrates).

- **Dinner:** Grilled tempeh (protein), steamed broccoli and carrots (vegetables and fruits), and a portion of brown rice (carbohydrates).

The Metabolic Plate Method simplifies your dietary approach while balancing all essential food groups. This supports weight management and metabolic health and encourages a healthy, varied, and enjoyable diet. With each meal, you can feel confident that you are nourishing your body effectively, helping you to maintain energy levels and avoid unnecessary snacking throughout the day.

Chapter 2:

CRAFTING A BALANCED DIET

Top 15 Plant-Based Sources of Vitamins and Minerals

1. **Chia Seeds (Calcium, Magnesium, Iron):** Their high fiber content helps stabilize blood sugar levels, making them ideal for people with diabetes. Omega-3 fatty acids and antioxidants may help prevent breast and colon cancer.

2. **Cabbage (Vitamin C, K, Manganese):** The low glycemic index suits people with diabetes. Sulforaphane and other antioxidants can prevent prostate, stomach, and colon cancer.

3. **Flaxseed (Magnesium, Iron, Vitamin B1):** Fiber helps control blood glucose, which benefits people with diabetes. Lignans protect against breast cancer.

4. **Blueberries (Vitamin C, Manganese, Vitamin K):** Their low glycemic index makes them a good choice for people with diabetes. Anthocyanins, powerful antioxidants, may reduce the risk of stomach and skin cancer.

5. **Brazil Nuts (Selenium, Magnesium):** Magnesium helps control blood sugar levels, which is essential for people with diabetes. Selenium has antioxidant properties that can protect against prostate and breast cancer.

6. **Spinach (Vitamins A, C, K, Magnesium, Iron):** Its high fiber content helps manage diabetes. Beta-carotene and other antioxidants can prevent skin, stomach, and lung cancer.

7. **Broccoli (Vitamins C, K, Calcium):** Rich in fiber, broccoli suits people with diabetes. Sulforaphane prevents prostate, breast, and colon cancer.

8. **Nuts, especially Almonds (Magnesium, Vitamin E, Calcium):** Maintain normal blood sugar levels. Vitamin E and other phytochemicals may reduce the risk of prostate and colon cancer.

9. **Pumpkin Seeds (Magnesium, Iron, Zinc):** Magnesium and fiber content help control diabetes. Phytoestrogens and zinc can protect against breast and prostate cancer.

10. **Quinoa (Magnesium, Phosphorus, Iron):** Complex carbohydrates with a low glycemic index maintain stable blood sugar levels, which benefits people with diabetes. Flavonoids and antioxidants may also reduce the risk of colon cancer.

11. **Avocado (Vitamins C, E, Potassium):** High in monounsaturated fats, helps control blood glucose levels, and improves insulin sensitivity. Thanks to their antioxidant properties, Vitamin E and beta-sitosterol may reduce the risk of prostate cancer.

12. **Peas (Vitamins C, K, Magnesium, and Iron):** Rich in fiber, which aids in the slow digestion of carbohydrates and maintains stable blood sugar levels. Antioxidants help reduce the risk of stomach and lung cancer by protecting cells from free radical damage.

13. **Sweet Potato (Vitamins A, C, Manganese):** A low glycemic index aids in maintaining stable blood sugar levels. Beta-carotene, a powerful antioxidant, is being studied for its ability to prevent pancreatic and colon cancer.

14. **Beans and Legumes (Iron, Zinc, Phosphorus, B Vitamins):** Their high fiber content helps control blood glucose and improve insulin sensitivity. Phytochemicals and fiber also help reduce the risk of colon cancer by preventing the formation of carcinogenic compounds in the intestine.

15. **Leafy Greens (Kale, Collard) (Vitamins A, C, K, Calcium):** Low-calorie and high in fiber, aiding in weight control and blood sugar regulation. High levels of vitamin C and other antioxidants can protect against colon and stomach cancer by neutralizing free radicals in tissues.

Protein Galore! Charting 150+ Plant-Based Protein Sources

This chapter provides a comprehensive guide to various protein-rich foods derived from plants. Each is carefully selected to enrich your diet with the necessary building blocks for a healthy body. From humble legumes to exotic seaweeds, from hearty grains to versatile nuts and seeds, we delve into the nutritional profiles that make each option a vital part of daily nourishment.

As we traverse meticulously curated tables—we illuminate each food's protein content and additional nutritional benefits. Highlighting indicators such as iron and calcium content, vitamin profiles, and amino acid completeness, these tables not only list foods but also the symbiotic relationships between their nutrients that are pivotal for optimal health.

This chapter will empower you with the knowledge and tools to construct a protein-rich menu. Protein is presented not as a mere nutrient but as a gateway to exploring the rich tapestry of plant-based eating, bringing together the essentials of taste, health, and sustainability.

Join me on this culinary journey as we unveil the robust world of plant-based proteins, a cornerstone for any modern diet that values health, diversity, and sustainability.

Key for Indicators:

IR: Rich in Iron

C: Contains Gluten
(Note: Fruits do not contain gluten unless contaminated.)

IC: Rich in Calcium

AA: Good Amino Acid Profile

B12: Sources of Vitamin B12

VD: Sources of Vitamin D

Top 20 Plant-Based Protein Champions per 100g: Dry Products in Case of Grains and Fresh Vegetables and Fruits

Product	Protein (g per 100g)	Indicators
Seitan	75	IR, C
Spirulina	57	IR, AA, B12, VD
Inactive Nutritional Yeast	40	AA, B12
Soy Flour	50	IR, AA, VD
Dried Nori	35	IC, B12, VD
Hemp Flour	33	AA, VD
Soy	36	IR, IC, AA, VD
Flaxseed Flour	32	IR, AA
Black Lentils	24	IR, AA
Hemp Seeds	31	IR, IC, AA
Sesame Burre	20	IC, AA
Hemp Seed Burre	30	IR, IC, AA
Pumpkin Seed Burre	30	IR, IC, AA
Peanut Burre	25	AA
Flaxseed Bran	25	AA
Peanuts	26	AA
Pumpkin Seeds	30	IR, IC, AA
Lentil Flour	28	IR, AA
Peanut Butter	25	AA
Apricot Kernel Burre	25	AA

Protein Content in Legumes and Grains per 100g: Dry Products in Case of Grains, and Fresh Vegetables and Fruits with Additional Nutrient Indicators

Product	Protein (g per 100g)	Indicators
Soy	36	IR, IC, AA, VD
Black Lentils	24	IR, AA
Red Lentils	27	IR, AA
Brown Lentils	25	IR, AA
Yellow Lentils	26	IR, AA
Mung Beans	24	IR, AA
Red Kidney Beans	24	IR, AA
Dried Peas	22	IR, AA
White Beans	21	IR, AA
Chickpeas	19	IR, AA
Fava Beans	26	IR, AA
Spelt	15	IR, C, IC
Oats	17	IR, C, IC, AA
Rye	15	IR, C, AA
Amaranth	14	IR, AA, VD
Black Rice	8	IR
Quinoa	14	IR, IC, AA, VD
Oat Flakes	13	IR, C, IC, AA
Bulgur	12	IR, C, AA
Buckwheat	13	IR, IC, AA
Wheat	12	IR, C, IC, AA
Couscous	15	IR, C, AA
Millet	11	IR, AA
Barley	12	IR, C, IC, AA
Pearl Barley	10	IR, C, IC, AA
Brown Rice	8	IR
Cornmeal	10	IR, AA
Polenta	10	IR, AA
Green Peas	5	IR, IC, AA

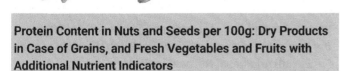

Protein Content in Nuts and Seeds per 100g: Dry Products in Case of Grains, and Fresh Vegetables and Fruits with Additional Nutrient Indicators

Product	Protein (g per 100g)	Indicators
Hemp Seeds	31	IR, AA
Peanuts	26	IR, AA
Pumpkin Seeds	30	IR, IC, AA
Pistachios	20	IR, AA
Apricot Kernels	25	IR, AA
Flax Seeds	18	IR, AA, VD
Cashews	18	IR, AA
Sunflower Seeds	21	IR, AA
Sesame Seeds	18	IR, IC, AA
Almonds	21	IR, AA
Chia Seeds	17	IR, AA, VD
Pine Nuts	14	IR, AA
Poppy Seeds	18	IR, CA, AA
Hazelnuts	15	IR, AA
Walnuts	15	IR, AA
Brazil Nuts	14	IR, AA, VD
Peeled Chestnuts	3	IR, IC
Pecans	9	IR, AA
Macadamia Nuts	8	IR, AA
Nutmeg	6	IR, AA
Coconut Flesh	3	IR

Protein Content in Flour, Pasta, and Bakery Products per 100g: Dry Products in Case of Grains, and Fresh Vegetables and Fruits with Additional Nutrient Indicators

Product	Protein (g per 100g)	Indicators
Soy Flour	50	IR, AA, VD
Hemp Flour	33	AA, VD
Linseed Flour	32	IR, AA
Linseed Bran	25	AA
Lentil Flour	28	IR, AA
Almond Flour	21	IR, AA
Chickpea Flour	22	IR, AA
Coconut Flour	18	IR, AA
Amaranth Bran	16	IR, AA, VD
Oat Bran	17	IR, C, IC, AA
Corn Bran	13	IR, AA
Wheat Bran	16	IR, C, AA
Buckwheat Bran	14	IR, AA
Rye Bran	15	IR, C, AA
Rice Bran	13	IR, AA
Buckwheat Flour	13	IR, IC, AA
Buckwheat Noodles	12	IR, AA
Pasta from Hard Wheat	13	IR, C, AA
Oat Flour	14	IR, C, AA
Barley Flour	12	IR, AA
Wheat Bread	10	C, AA
Wheat Flour	11	IR, C, AA
Rye Flour	15	IR, C, AA
Corn Flour	8	IR, AA
Rye Bread	9	IR, C, AA
Rice Flour	7	IR, AA
Rice Noodles	4	IR

Protein Content in Butter per 100g: Dry Products in Case of Grains, and Fresh Vegetables and Fruits with Additional Nutrient Indicators

Product	Protein (g per 100g)	Indicators
Hemp Seed Butter	30	IR, AA
Pumpkin Seed Butter	30	IR, AA
Sesame Butter	20	IR, IC, AA
Peanut Butter	25	AA
Peanut Paste	25	AA
Apricot Kernel Butter	25	AA
Cashew Butter	18	AA
Flax Seed Butter	18	IR, AA
Almond Butter	21	IR, AA
Sunflower Seed Butter	20	IR, AA
Pistachio Butter	20	IR, AA
Poppy Seed Butter	18	IR, CA, AA
Hazelnut Butter	15	IR, AA
Walnut Butter	15	IR, AA

Protein Content in Mushrooms per 100g: Dry Products in Case of Grains, and Fresh Vegetables and Fruits with Additional Nutrient Indicators

Mushroom Type	Protein (g per 100g)	Indicators
White Button Mushrooms	3.1	AA
Cremini Mushrooms	2.5	AA
Portobello Mushrooms	2.1	AA
Shiitake Mushrooms	2.2	IR, AA
Oyster Mushrooms	3.3	IR, AA
Enoki Mushrooms	2.7	AA
Morel Mushrooms	3.1	IR, AA

Protein Content in Vegetables and Seaweeds per 100g: Dry Products in Case of Grains, and Fresh Vegetables and Fruits with Additional Nutrient Indicators

Product	Protein (g per 100g)	Indicators
Dried Nori	35	IR, IC, B12, VD
Dried Wakame	20	IR, IC, B12, VD
Fresh Wakame	3	IR, IC, B12, VD
Chuka Seaweed	5	IR, IC, AA, VD
Kale	4.3	IR, IC, AA, VD
Broccoli	2.8	IR, IC, AA, VD
Spinach	2.9	IR, IC, AA, VD
Brussels Sprouts	3.4	IR, IC, AA, VD
Green Beans	1.8	IR, AA
Asparagus	2.2	IR, AA
Parsley	3.0	IR, IC, AA
Dill	2.5	IR, IC, AA
Garlic	6.4	IR, AA
Leeks	1.5	IR, AA
Basil	3.2	IR, AA
Cilantro	2.1	IR, AA
Horseradish	2.0	IR, AA
Yellow Onion	1.1	AA
Carrots	0.9	AA
Radish	0.6	AA
Sweet Potato	1.6	AA
Corn	3.2	AA
Potato	2.0	AA
Pumpkin	1.0	AA

Protein Content in Plant-Based Milks per 100g: Dry Products in Case of Grains, and Fresh Vegetables and Fruits with Additional Nutrient Indicators

Plant Milk	Protein (g per 100g)	Indicators
Soy Milk	3.3	IR, IC, AA, B12, VD
Oat Milk	0.5	IC, VD
Almond Milk	0.5	IR, AA
Coconut Milk	0.5	IR
Pine Nut Milk	1.0	IR, AA

Protein Content in Fruits and Dried Fruits per 100g: Dry Products in Case of Grains, and Fresh Vegetables and Fruits with Additional Nutrient Indicators

Fruit/Dried Fruit	Protein (g per 100g)	Indicators
Dried Apricots	3.4	IR
Dried Figs	3.3	IR
Raisins	3.1	IR
Prunes	2.2	IR, AA
Dates	2.5	IR
Guava	2.6	IR, IC, AA
Passion Fruit	2.2	IR, IC
Blackcurrant	1.4	IR, IC, AA
Avocado	2.0	IR, IC, AA
Durian	1.5	IR
Banana	1.1	IR
Blackberries	1.4	IR, AA
Apricot	1.4	IR
Raspberry	1.2	IR, AA
Kiwi	1.1	IR, IC, AA

Protein Content in Other Foods per 100g: Dry Products in Case of Grains, and Fresh Vegetables and Fruits with Additional Nutrient Indicators

Product	Protein (g per 100g)	Indicators
Seitan	75	C, AA
Spirulina	57	IR, AA, B12, VD
Nutritional Yeast (Deactivated)	40	B12, AA
Tempeh	19	IR, AA
Tofu (Firm)	8	IR, IC, AA
Dark Chocolate	7.6	IR
Soft Tofu	5	IR, IC, AA
Cocoa	20	IR, AA
Carob	4.6	IR, IC
Tomato Paste	4.3	IR, IC, AA, VD

Fermentation: The Secret Path to Amino Acids, Vitamins, and Minerals. How a Plant-Based Diet Transforms Us and Our Microbiota

The Gut: The Mysterious Garden of Health and a Plant-Based Diet

Scientists have discovered that our gut is not just an organ but a whole cosmos of microbes. Microbes are closely linked to diseases like diabetes, obesity, autoimmune disorders, and even mental health.

A plant-based diet is like an elite health club. It is like a VIP party for our microbiota. The fiber and polyphenols we get from plants are like exclusive drinks and snacks for our microbial friends. They thrive, and our chances of living a healthy life increase.

Taking care of your gut is taking care of yourself. Your gut will thank you after switching to a plant-based diet. Expect reduced inflammation, improved digestion, and a better mood - all bonuses of embracing a plant-based diet. It's also a great conversation starter with your friends about your new culinary exploration!

Vitamin B12, Muscle Mass, and Human Gut Microbiota: What's the Connection?

What concerns do fans of a plant-based diet, especially vegans, have? Naturally, the main issues are often the potential for protein deficiency and a lack of vitamin B12. However, nature is on our side, and understanding the processes that form our bodies and the ability to absorb nutrients is crucial. Our gut flora is diverse and directly dependent on the food we consume. This flora can synthesize amino acids to build our body, and even in the gut, there's potential for additional synthesis of vitamin B12, thanks to certain bacteria. An underappreciated category in human diets is fermented products. Often overlooked, regular consumption of fermented products can significantly enhance our gut microbiota.

Fermentation enhances flavor, extends shelf life, and increases nutritional value. Here are some examples of plant-based fermented products:

1. Sauerkraut is cabbage fermented with various lactic acid bacteria and is a rich source of vitamins C and K, as well as probiotics.

2. Kimchi is a traditional Korean dish usually made from fermented cabbage with various spices and seasonal vegetables. It is known for its probiotic properties.

3. Tempeh is a soy-based product fermented with Rhizopus mold. It is rich in protein, B vitamins, and numerous minerals.

4. Miso is a Japanese paste from fermented soybeans, salt, and rice or barley koji. It is rich in proteins, vitamin K, and various minerals.

5. Kombucha is a fermented tea produced by a symbiosis of bacteria and yeast. This drink is known for its detoxification and energy-boosting properties.

6. Soy sauce is made from fermented soybeans, wheat, water, and salt. It is rich in amino acids formed during fermentation.

These plant-based fermented products diversify the diet and significantly contribute to gut health thanks to the probiotics that support the balance of gut flora. They can also aid in improving digestion and nutrient absorption.

Some fermented products can be bought in a regular health food store, and others can be made at home. The most straightforward and accessible recipe is for fermented cabbage. I share an easy way to prepare this dish later.

The Beneficial Aspects of a Plant-Based Diet with Fermented Products for Humans:

1. **Improved Digestion:** Fermented products contain probiotics, which are live microorganisms that promote gut health. These microorganisms can aid in digesting plant food, increasing nutrient assimilation efficiency, and improving the gut microbiota's overall condition.

2. **Enhanced Nutrient Absorption:** Plants contain many vitamins, minerals, and antioxidants. Fermentation increases the bioavailability of these nutrients, making them more digestible for the human body, similar to how microbes in the rumen help ruminants absorb nutrients from plants.

3. **Immune System Support:** A healthy gut microbiota is linked to a strong immune system. Enriched with probiotics, fermented products can help maintain a balance of beneficial intestinal bacteria, improving immune function.

4. **Disease Prevention:** Just as ruminants derive nutrients from plants to maintain health and prevent diseases, a plant-based diet with fermented products can help prevent numerous diseases, including cardiovascular diseases, type 2 diabetes, and certain cancers, due to improved nutrition and gut health.

How often should you consume fermented products? The answer is unequivocal: the more frequently, the better. Aim for daily if you can. Besides their immense benefits, they're also flavor bombs for your dishes. Take fermented vegetables like cabbage. Their tangy kick adds a new dimension to plant-based burgers or tacos, without needing extra salt. The left-over brine is also a gut-loving elixir packed with vitamins.

Want to go deeper into the world of ferments? Check out *"Wild Fermentation: The Flavor, Nutrition, and Craft of Live-Culture Foods"* by Sandor Ellix Katz. If you are keen to explore the magic of fermentation, this book will be handy for you.

Date-Sweetened Vegan Kimchi

Prep Time: 45 minutes, Servings: 8

INGREDIENTS:

1 large Napa cabbage (about 2.2 lbs or 1 kg)

4 tbsp coarse sea salt

1-2 tbsp date puree (adjust sweetness to taste)

3 cloves garlic, finely minced

1-inch piece ginger, finely minced

1 small daikon radish, julienned

2 tbsp Korean red pepper paste (gochujang)

1/2 cup Korean red pepper flakes (gochugaru)

3 green onions, chopped

2 tbsp soy sauce or tamari (for a gluten-free option)

1 tbsp sesame seeds for garnish

INSTRUCTIONS:

1. **Prepare the Cabbage:** Cut the cabbage in half lengthwise, then slice each half into quarters. Remove the cores and sprinkle each layer with salt. Let the cabbage sit for 2 hours, turning every 30 minutes to ensure even salting.

2. **Make the Paste:** Combine the date puree, minced garlic, ginger, soy sauce, and gochujang in a small bowl. Stir until well mixed.

3. **Mix Vegetables:** Rinse the salted cabbage under cold water thoroughly and drain. Combine the cabbage with the radish and green onions in a large mixing bowl.

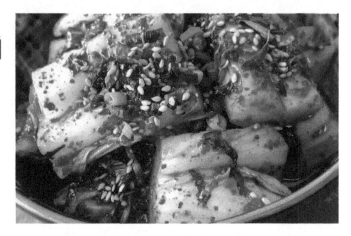

Add the prepared paste and mix well, preferably with gloves to protect your hands.

4. **Fermentation:** Pack the kimchi into a clean glass jar, pressing down to remove air pockets. Seal the jar and leave it at room temperature for 1-2 days for initial fermentation. Then, store it in the refrigerator for at least one week before eating.

5. **Serve:** Enjoy chilled, garnished with sesame seeds. Kimchi can be stored in the refrigerator for 2-3 months.

Cooking Method: No cooking. Fermentation.

NUTRITIONAL INFORMATION
(APPROXIMATE PER SERVING, ABOUT 1/2 CUP):

Calories: 70 kcal | Protein: 2 g | Fat: 1 g | Carb: 14 g | Fiber: 3 g

---

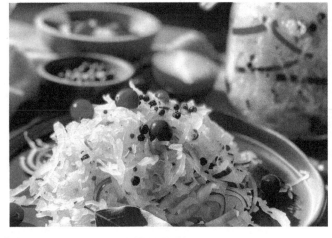

NUTRITIONAL INFORMATION
(APPROXIMATE PER SERVING):

Calories: 30-35 kcal | Protein: 1.5 g | Fat: 0.1 g | Carb: 7 g | Fiber: 3 g

STORAGE:

Store between 0°C and 4°C (32°F-39°F).

Avoid metal containers or utensils.

Homemade Fermentation of Cabbage (Sauerkraut)

Prep Time: 30 min (plus 4 days fermentation), Servings: ~10

INGREDIENTS:

0.5 liters water

1.5 kg cabbage

200 g carrots

15-22 g sea salt (1-1.5% of total vegetable weight)

INSTRUCTIONS:

1. **Shred & Salt:** Shred the cabbage and carrots. Sprinkle with sea salt and mix. Let sit for 15-20 minutes to release juices.

2. **Pack & Cover:** Pack the vegetables into a glass or ceramic container, ensuring they're submerged in liquid. Add water if needed.

3. **Ferment:** Cover with a towel and lid. Ferment at room temperature for 4 days, releasing gas daily by poking the mixture.

4. **Store:** After 4 days, seal and refrigerate.

The Sprout Revolution: Harnessing the Power of Microgreens to Supercharge Dishes with Vitamins and Minerals

Sprouts are more than just a trendy ingredient for smoothies and salads; they are a whole universe of nutrients. These little green wonders are the unique superheroes of nutrition.

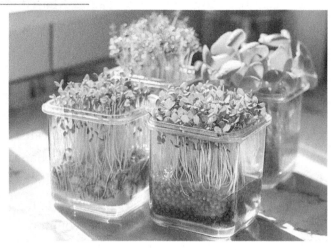

Growing sprouts at home is a particular pleasure. A micro garden is an ideal fit for your kitchen. Try it— it's straightforward, and you'll have a harvest in just a few days. Sprouts also give you aesthetic pleasure and inspiration by decorating your kitchen with delicate shoots.

Most Beneficial Types of Sprouts

Alfalfa – a star among sprouts. Rich in vitamins K, C, and trace elements.

Broccoli – these guys are real fighters against antioxidants.

Peas – an excellent source of protein and fiber.

Wheat – a treasure trove of magnesium and iron and is also great for improving digestion.

Radish – a real vitamin explosion, especially rich in vitamin C.

Vitamin Composition and Effect on the Body

Vitamins: Vitamin C (for immunity), vitamin K (for bones), vitamin E (antioxidant), and B vitamins (energy metabolism).

Minerals: Iron (against anemia), magnesium (for the nervous system), calcium (for bones).

Phytonutrients: Sulforaphane (in broccoli, a powerful antioxidant).

Protein: Essential in vegetarian and vegan diets.

Consumption

Sprouts are versatile. They can be added to smoothies, salads, and sandwiches. To keep their health benefits intact, it's best to enjoy them lightly steamed.

In the United States, ready-made sprouts can be purchased at various grocery stores, including Sprouts Farmers Market, known for its wide range of healthy, organic, and fresh produce. Other major grocery stores like Whole Foods often stock a variety of sprouts, and they are known for their emphasis on natural and organic foods. You can find sprouts in these stores among the fresh produce sections.

The Theory of 5 Tastes: Balancing Flavors for Maximum Delight

As we explore the diverse world of a plant-based diet, let's explore the incredible world of flavor it offers. Our taste buds naturally crave different sensations, from savory to sweet. Understanding this connection between biology and psychology is key to creating tasty and satisfying plant-based meals.

So, why are we attracted to certain flavors, such as salty or sweet? Essentially, our bodies are biochemically tuned to seek out flavors that signal specific nutrients necessary for survival. Salt, for example, indicates the presence of minerals. Sweet often indicates energy-rich sugars. Meanwhile, our penchant for fried foods can be explained by their high-calorie content, which provides a dense energy source that our ancestors rarely encountered and, therefore, from an evolutionary perspective, needs to be utilized when available.

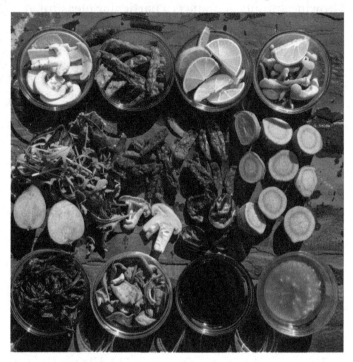

The connection between our brain and our taste buds is complex. When food hits our taste buds, signals are sent to the brain that activate reward pathways and release neurotransmitters, such as dopamine, that enhance the pleasure and satisfaction derived from food. This biological circuitry explains why certain foods are more addictive and why cravings for them are common in humans.

A balance of these flavors can transform plant-based food from ordinary to delicious. The key is to combine elements of each flavor, allowing them to harmonize and enhance the dish's overall taste.

Plant foods abound with these flavors if you know where to look.

Sweet: Sweetness satisfies our desire for something pleasurable and provides us with energy. In a plant-based diet, find it in fruits such as bananas, apples, mangoes, and dates and vegetables such as corn, red bell peppers, pumpkin, sweet potatoes, carrots, and beets.

Salty: These flavors help fulfil our mineral requirements and can add depth to a dish. Green leafy vegetables such as spinach and chard naturally contain sodium. Seaweed, including nori and dulse, is a rich source of salty flavor. Soy sauce or tamari can add saltiness to sauces and marinades.

Sour: Sour tastes can refresh and enhance any dish by adding brightness. Citrus fruits, including lemons, limes, and grapefruit are great sources. Vinegars such as apple, balsamic, and rice also bring sourness, as do fermented foods such as kimchi, sauerkraut and tempeh.

Bitter: These flavors are often associated with detoxification and can complicate the flavor profile. Green leafy vegetables, including kale, arugula, radicchio, and herbs such as cola, chicory, wild spinach, coffee, and cocoa, also have a natural bitterness.

Umami: Adds richness and depth to dishes, which is especially important in plant-based diets. Mushrooms like shiitake and portobello bring an earthy depth. Ripe tomatoes, especially if slightly dried, add a concentrated burst of flavor. Nutritional yeast, soy sauce, and miso add a rich umami punch.

The variety of these products makes it easy to incorporate different flavors into your plant-based diet, making each meal unique and satisfying. It takes a lot of work to embrace all five flavors in one meal.

Let's make things easy with sauces that combine all five flavors. This small addition to a main dish will give a palette of sensations and satiety. These sauces combine complex flavors that make every bite hearty and enrich your plant-based dishes with depth and excitement.

Spicy ginger and turmeric sauce

Prep Time: 5 minutes
Servings: Approximately 1/2 cup (about 8 tablespoons)

INGREDIENTS:

2 tbsp freshly grated ginger

1 tsp turmeric powder

Juice of 1 lemon

1 tbsp soy sauce

2 tbsp sesame oil

1 tbsp agave syrup or date puree

A pinch of black pepper (to activate the turmeric)

NUTRITIONAL INFORMATION
(APPROXIMATE PER TABLESPOON):

Calories: 25-30 kcal | Protein: 0.3 g | Fat: 2 g | Carbohydrates: 2 g | Fiber: 0.2 g

INSTRUCTIONS:

Combine all ingredients in a blender and chop until smooth.

Cashew cream with lime and cilantro

Prep Time: 15 minutes (plus 4 hours soaking time)
Servings: Approximately 1 cup (about 8 tablespoons)

INGREDIENTS:

1 cup raw cashews soaked for 4 hours and drained

Juice of 2 limes

1/4 cup fresh cilantro, chopped

1 tsp garlic powder

2 tbsp nutritional yeast

Himalayan salt, if desired

Water to adjust consistency

NUTRITIONAL INFORMATION
(APPROXIMATE PER TABLESPOON):

Calories: 50-55 kcal | Protein: 2 g | Fat: 4 g | Carb: 3 g | Fiber: 0.5 g

INSTRUCTIONS:

Place all ingredients in a high-speed blender until smooth and creamy. Add water as needed to achieve the desired thickness. This creamy sauce is perfect for sprinkling over tacos or as a dip for crispy potato wedges.

Spicy Carrot-Ginger Sauce

Prep Time: 15 minutes
Servings: 1 cup (approximately 8 tablespoons)

INGREDIENTS:

2 large carrots, cooked until soft

2 inches grated fresh ginger

1 tbsp miso paste

1 tbsp tahini

1/4 tsp cinnamon

1 tbsp maple syrup or some mashed dates

2 tbsp lemon juice

Himalayan salt, if desired

Mixing water

NUTRITIONAL INFORMATION
(APPROXIMATE PER TABLESPOON):

Calories: 20-25 kcal | Protein: 0.5 g | Fat: 1 g | Carb: 3 g | Fiber: 1 g

INSTRUCTIONS:

Combine all ingredients in a blender and chop until smooth. This vibrant sauce is excellent with roasted vegetables or as a flavorful base for a vegetable-based soup.

Roasted Red Peppers and Almond Pesto

Prep Time: 15 minutes
Servings: Approximately 1 cup (about 8 servings)

INGREDIENTS:

1 cup roasted red peppers (about two large peppers)

1/2 cup raw almonds

1 clove garlic

1/4 cup basil leaves

2 tbsp nutritional yeast

Juice of 1/2 lemon

Salt and pepper to taste as desired

Olive oil to achieve the desired consistency

NUTRITIONAL INFORMATION
(APPROXIMATE PER TABLESPOON):

Calories: 35-45 kcal | Protein: 1 g | Fat: 3 g | Carb: 2 g | Fiber: 1 g

INSTRUCTIONS:

In a food processor, blend roasted peppers, almonds, garlic, basil, and nutritional yeast until coarsely ground. While processing, gradually add olive oil and lemon juice until the pesto has the desired texture. Season with salt and pepper. This pesto is great with pasta, spread on sandwiches, or added to grains for flavor.

Spicy Ginger and Sesame Sauce

Prep Time: 5 minutes
Servings: Approximately 1/2 cup (about 8 tablespoons)

INGREDIENTS:

2 tbsp toasted sesame oil

1 tbsp finely grated ginger

2 tbsp soy sauce

2 tbsp rice vinegar

1 tsp agave syrup or some mashed dates

1 tsp sesame seeds for decoration

NUTRITIONAL INFORMATION
(APPROXIMATE PER TABLESPOON):

Calories: 30-35 kcal | Protein: 0.5 g | Fat: 3 g | Carb: 1 g | Fiber: 0.2 g

INSTRUCTIONS:

In a small bowl, mix the sesame oil, grated ginger, soy sauce, rice vinegar, and agave syrup or mashed dates until smooth. Before serving, sprinkle sesame seeds on top. This sauce is excellent for salad dressing, spring rolls, and Asian-style dishes.

Substituting Familiar Ingredients

Switching to a plant-based diet isn't about giving up your favorite flavors and textures. It's about finding creative and satisfying alternatives that align with healthier and more sustainable eating habits. In this chapter, we'll look at replacing familiar ingredients with plant-based options to keep the essence of your favorite dishes.

- **Beef/Pork:** For recipes calling for ground beef or pork, consider using lentils, textured vegetable protein (TVP), or finely chopped mushrooms. These alternatives provide a meaty texture and perfectly absorb flavors.

- **Chicken:** Jackfruit, particularly canned young green jackfruit in water, is a great substitute for chicken due to its texture.Seitan and tofu are also great for imitating chicken pieces in stir-fries and curries.

- **Milk:** Almond, soy, oat, and cashew milk are popular dairy-free alternatives.

- **Cheese:** Nutritional yeast can impart a cheesy flavor to popcorn or pasta, and cashew cheese is creamy and versatile enough for spreads and sauces. Store-bought vegan cheeses offer a wide variety of textures and flavors.

- **Butter:** Coconut oil can be a direct substitute for butter in baking, or you can use vegan products whose flavor and texture are similar to dairy butter.

- **Egg for baking:** Replace one egg with one tablespoon of ground flaxseed mixed with three tablespoons of water and let stand until it becomes gelatinous. Applesauce or banana puree is also suitable for cakes and muffins.

- **Preparation:** Tofu omelets are a fantastic eggless alternative. Add turmeric for a natural egg-like color and black salt to mimic the sulfuric flavor of eggs.

- **Fish:** Nori or other seaweed can give dishes a fishy flavor. Palm kernel or artichoke hearts can mimic the texture of fish flakes in salads and cakes.

- **Shellfish:** Royal oyster mushrooms have a chewy texture suitable for replacing scallops. Jackfruit can be used as a substitute in recipes calling for crabmeat, especially if seasoned appropriately.

- **Sugars:** Dates, maple syrup, and coconut sugar are great alternatives to naturally sweetening dishes. They also contain additional nutrients not found in refined sugar.

- **Animal Fats for cooking.** Instead of lard or butter, choose avocado oil, olive oil, or other vegetable oils.

- **Traditional pasta:** Substitutes such as lentils, chickpeas, or zucchini noodles (zoodles) contain more fiber and protein than regular pasta.

- **White rice:** Quinoa, cauliflower rice, and barley are nutritious substitutes that provide additional health benefits such as more protein and fiber.

- **Salt Dried Tomato Powder:** This powder is a concentrated source of umami and saltiness. Dried tomatoes have a deep flavor, which makes them an excellent addition to sauces, soups, and casseroles.

- **Dried Celery powder:** Dried celery powder contains natural sodium and can add a salty flavor without salt. It is a great way to enhance the flavor of various dishes, especially soups and meat preparations.

- **Lemon or lime juice:** The acidity of these citrus fruits can enhance the flavor of food, intensify the effect, and add saltiness. This works exceptionally well in salads and seafood.

- **Vinegar:** Apple or wine vinegar can add an acidic taste to dishes and enhance their flavor by replacing some of the salt.

- **Herbs and spices:** Fresh or dried herbs (such as rosemary, thyme, and basil) and spices (such as black pepper, chili, and turmeric) can significantly enhance the flavor of dishes, thus reducing the need for salt. Specialties such as Italian seasoning or curries are also a great choice.

- **Miso paste:** This fermented soybean paste adds depth and complexity to dishes, allowing you to cut back on added salt.

- **Nutritional Yeast Extract (nutritional yeast):** This product is rich in umami and can impart cheesy and salty flavors without adding salt. It is perfect for vegetarian and vegan dishes.

- **Black salt (kala namak):** Although it is still salt, it has a unique flavor reminiscent of the taste of eggs. It can be an exciting alternative to vegan dishes such as vegan omelets.

- **Fermented vegetables:** Kimchi, cucumbers, or sauerkraut can add a distinct flavor and salt to dishes.

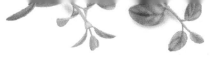

Chapter 3:

BREAKFASTS

POWER-PACKED PROTEIN SMOOTHIES

Tropical Mango-Turmeric Smoothie

Prep Time: 5 minutes, Servings: 1-2

INGREDIENTS:

- 1 cup of mango (can be fresh or frozen)
- 1 small banana
- 1/2 cup pineapple (can be fresh or frozen)
- 1 tsp turmeric
- 1 cup coconut milk
- 2. tbsp shredded coconut
- 1 tbsp chia seeds

INSTRUCTIONS:

Place all ingredients in a blender. Blend on high speed until smooth and creamy. Pour the smoothie into a glass and, if desired, garnish with additional shredded coconut on top.

Cooking Method: No cooking. Blending.

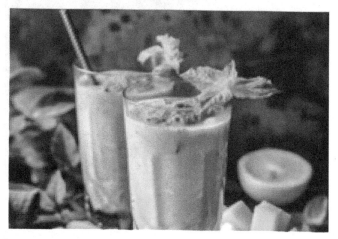

NUTRITIONAL INFORMATION
(APPROXIMATE PER SERVING):

Calories: 350 kcal | Carbs: 50 g | Fat: 15 g | Fiber: 8 g | Cholesterol: 0 mg | Sodium: 50 mg

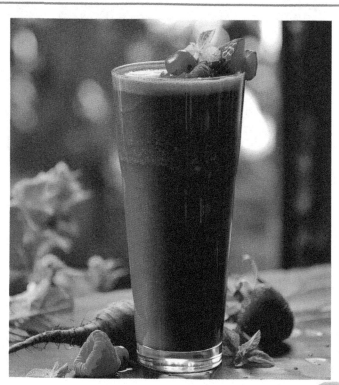

Berry-Beet Energizer Smoothie

Preparation Time: 5 minutes, Servings: 1-2

INGREDIENTS:

- 1/2 beet, chopped
- 1 cup mixed berries (raspberries, strawberries; can be fresh or frozen)
- 1 banana
- 1 cup almond milk
- 1 tbsp flax seeds

INSTRUCTIONS:

Place all ingredients in a blender. Blend on high speed until smooth. Serve the smoothie immediately, and enjoy the fresh and energizing taste.

Cooking Method: No cooking. Blending.

NUTRITIONAL INFORMATION
(APPROXIMATE PER SERVING):

Calories: 300 kcal | Carbs: 50 g | Fat: 7 g | Fiber: 9 g | Cholesterol: 0 mg | Sodium: 95 mg

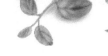

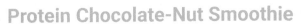

Protein Chocolate-Nut Smoothie

Prep Time: 5 minutes, Servings:1-2

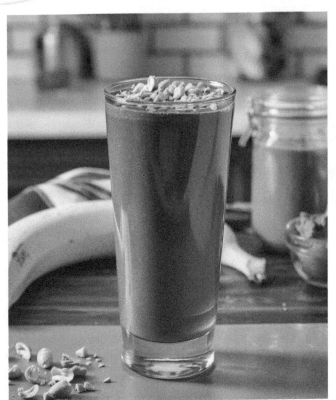

INGREDIENTS:

2 tbsp cocoa powder

1 banana

1 cup nut milk (cashew or almond)

1 tbsp peanut butter

1 tbsp flax seeds

INSTRUCTIONS:

Add all ingredients to a blender. Blend on high until smooth and creamy. Pour into a glass and serve immediately for a protein-rich treat.

Cooking Method: No cooking. Blending.

NUTRITIONAL INFORMATION (APPROXIMATE PER SERVING):

Calories: 320 kcal | Carbs: 40 g | Fat: 16 g | Fiber: 7 g | Cholesterol: 0 mg | Sodium: 150 mg

Antioxidant Blueberry-Spinach Smoothie

PrepTime: 5 minutes, Servings: 1-2

INGREDIENTS:

1 cup frozen blueberries

1 cup fresh spinach

1 banana

1 cup coconut water

1 tbsp flax seeds

INSTRUCTIONS:

Combine all ingredients in a blender. Blend on high until smooth and uniform in texture. Serve the smoothie immediately, enjoying its refreshing and healthful benefits.

Cooking Method: No cooking. Blending.

NUTRITIONAL INFORMATION (APPROXIMATE PER SERVING):

Calories: 280 kcal | Carbs: 53 g | Fat: 4 g | Fiber: 8 g | Cholesterol: 0 mg | Sodium: 70 mg

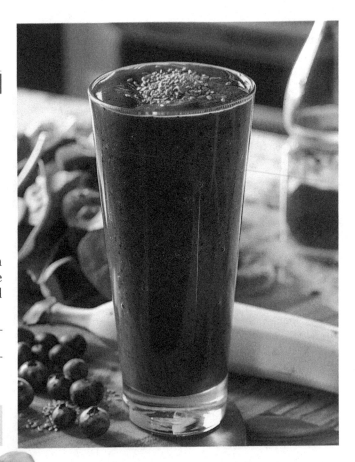

Green Energy Smoothie

INGREDIENTS:

1 cup curly kale

1 green apple, chopped

1/2 an avocado

Juice of 1 lime

1 cup almond milk

INSTRUCTIONS:

Place kale, green apple, avocado, and lime juice in a blender. Add almond milk to the blender. Blend all ingredients on high until smooth. Pour into a glass and serve immediately for a burst of green energy.

Cooking Method: No cooking. Blending.

NUTRITIONAL INFORMATION (APPROXIMATE PER SERVING):

Calories: 240 kcal | Carbs: 30 g | Fat: 15 g | Fiber: 6 g | Cholesterol: 0 mg | Sodium: 95 mg

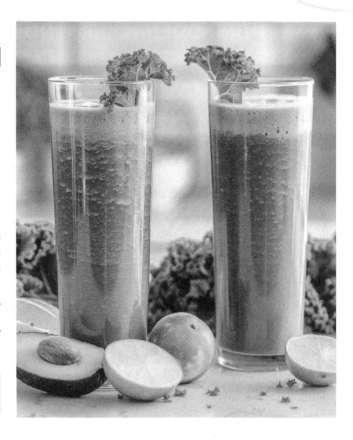

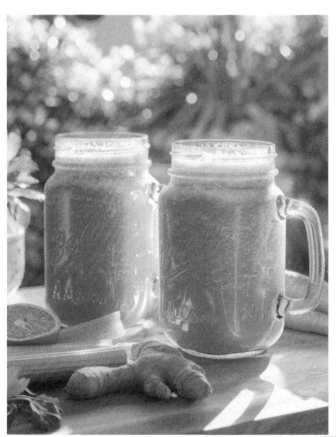

Celery and Carrot Smoothie

Prep: 5 minutes, Servings: 1-2

INGREDIENTS:

3 celery stalks, chopped

2 carrots, chopped

Juice of 1 orange

1/2 tsp ginger root, chopped

1 cup of water

INSTRUCTIONS:

Add celery, carrots, orange juice, and ginger root to a blender. Pour water into the blender. Blend all ingredients on high until smooth. Serve the smoothie immediately; it is refreshing and nutritious.

Cooking Method: No cooking. Blending.

NUTRITIONAL INFORMATION (APPROXIMATE PER SERVING):

Calories: 150 kcal | Carbs: 35 g | Fat: 0.5 g | Fiber: 8 g | Cholesterol: 0 mg | Sodium: 125 mg

PORRIDGES - QUICK, NUTRITIOUS, AND ENERGIZING

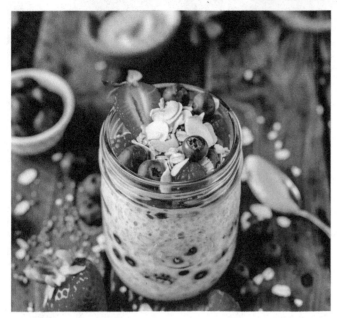

Apple Cinnamon Bircher Muesli

Prep Time: 10 minutes + overnight soaking, Servings: 2

INGREDIENTS:

1 cup rolled oats

3/4 cup natural apple puree

1/2 cup plant-based milk (almond or oat)

2 medium apples, grated

1/2 tsp ground cinnamon

1/4 cup chopped nuts (walnuts or almonds)

Optional: Seeds (flaxseeds or chia)

INSTRUCTIONS:

1. **Preparation:** Mix oats and apple puree in a bowl, cover, and refrigerate overnight.

2. **Mixing:** In the morning, stir in plant-based milk, grated apple, and cinnamon. Add nuts and seeds if desired.

3. **Serving:** Top with fresh apple slices, nuts, and a sprinkle of cinnamon.

NUTRITIONAL INFORMATION (APPROXIMATE PER SERVING):

Calories: 320 | Protein: 6g | Fat: 10g | Carbs: 54g | Fiber: 8g

---

Raw Energy Breakfast Bowl

Prep Time: Overnight soaking, Servings: 2

INGREDIENTS:

2 tbsp flax seeds

2 tbsp chia seeds

1 tbsp raw sesame seeds

2 tbsp nuts (almonds, pecans, hazelnuts, or cashews)

2 tbsp dried cherries (or raisins, apricots, prunes, chopped)

2 cups cold water

Optional: 1 banana for blending

INSTRUCTIONS:

1. **Combine:** Mix flax, chia, sesame seeds, nuts, and dried fruit in a bowl.

2. **Soak:** Add 2 cups water, stir, cover, and refrigerate overnight.

3. **Blend:** In the morning, transfer to a blender; add a banana for creaminess, if desired.

4. **Serve:** Blend until smooth. Enjoy chilled or gently warmed on the stove (below 118°F to retain nutrients).

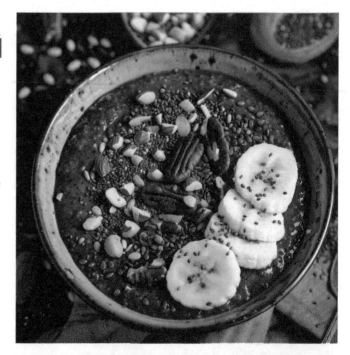

NUTRITION PER SERVING (WITHOUT BANANA):

Calories: 275 | Protein: 8g | Fat: 15g | Carbs: 30g | Fiber: 9g

OMELETS: REVOLUTIONIZING THE CLASSICS

Tofu Omelet with Spinach and Tomatoes

Cooking Time: 20 minutes, Servings: 2

INGREDIENTS:

- 200 g tofu, pressed and crumbled
- 1 tbsp nutritional yeast
- 1/4 tsp turmeric
- 1/2 tsp black pepper
- 1 tsp Himalayan salt
- 1/2 cup water
- 1 tbsp olive oil
- 1/2 cup fresh spinach
- 1 medium tomato, diced
- 2 tbsp green onions, chopped

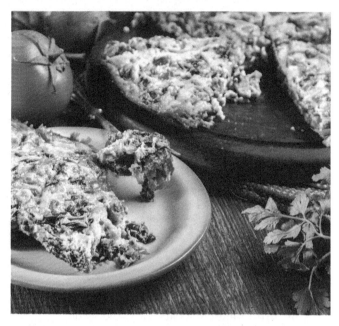

INSTRUCTIONS:

1. **Mix:** In a bowl, combine tofu, nutritional yeast, turmeric, black pepper, salt, and water until smooth.

2. **Cook:** Heat olive oil in a pan over medium. Add tofu mixture, spreading it evenly. Top with spinach, tomatoes, and green onions. Cook for 5-7 minutes until golden on the bottom, then flip and cook for 3-4 more minutes.

NUTRITION PER SERVING:

Calories: 180 | Protein: 12g | Fat: 10g | Carbs: 8g

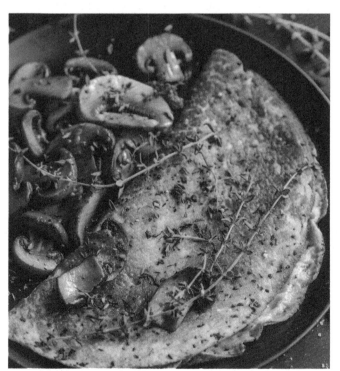

Chickpea Flour Omelet with Mushrooms and Thyme

Cooking Time: 25 minutes, Servings: 2

INGREDIENTS:

- 1/2 cup chickpea flour
- 1 tsp nutritional yeast
- 1/2 tsp celery salt
- 1 tbsp olive oil
- 1 cup mushrooms, chopped
- 1/4 tsp dried thyme
- 1 cup almond milk (or other plant-based milk)

INSTRUCTIONS:

1. **Mix:** Combine chickpea flour, nutritional yeast, celery salt, and almond milk in a bowl until smooth.

2. **Cook Mushrooms:** Heat olive oil in a skillet, add mushrooms and thyme, and cook until tender, about 5 minutes.

3. **Add Chickpea Mix:** Pour chickpea mixture over mushrooms. Cook on low until golden on the bottom, then flip and cook for a few more minutes.

NUTRITION PER SERVING:

Calories: 220 | Protein: 9g | Fat: 12g | Carbs: 18g

HOMEMADE MUESLI: CRAFTING THE PERFECT START

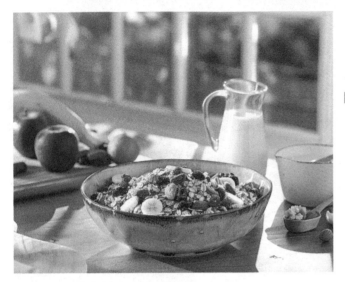

Ultimate Muesli Medley: Sunrise Symphony & Morning Bliss

Prep Time: 20 minutes, Servings: 6 per variant

BASE INGREDIENTS:

6 cups rolled oats

1 1/2 cups chopped raw nuts

3/4 cup sunflower or pumpkin seeds

Optional: 1/2 cup applesauce, 3/4 cup chia seeds

Variants:

Sunrise Symphony: 1/4 cup coconut, 1/2 cup dried fruit, 1 tsp cinnamon, 1/4 tsp salt

Morning Bliss: 1/4 cup carob powder, 1/4 cup cacao nibs, 1/2 tsp vanilla, 1/4 tsp salt

INSTRUCTIONS:

1. **Combine Base:** Mix oats, nuts, and seeds.
2. **Divide:** Separate into two bowls, add ingredients for each variant:
   - Sunrise Symphony: Coconut, dried fruit, cinnamon, salt.
   - Morning Bliss: Carob, cacao nibs, vanilla, salt.
3. **Optional Binding:** Add applesauce and chia if desired.

NUTRITION PER SERVING:

Calories: 250-300 | Protein: 6-8g | Fat: 10-15g | Carbs: 30-40g | Fiber: 5-7g

Autumn Essence Energy Bars

Cooking Time: 30 minutes, Servings: 12

INGREDIENTS:

1 cup rolled oats

1/2 cup chopped almonds (or mixed nuts)

1/2 cup chopped walnuts

1/4 cup pumpkin seeds

1/4 cup sunflower seeds

1/2 cup dried cranberries

1/2 cup chopped apricots

1/4 cup raisins

2 tbsp flaxseeds + 6 tbsp water

1/2 cup date puree

1 tsp vanilla

1/2 tsp cinnamon

INSTRUCTIONS:

1. **Preheat Oven:** To 350°F (175°C). Line an 8x8-inch dish.
2. **Prepare Flax:** Mix flaxseed with water; let thicken.
3. **Mix Dry:** Combine oats, nuts, seeds, dried fruit, and cinnamon.
4. **Blend Dates:** Make a thick puree with dates and minimal water.

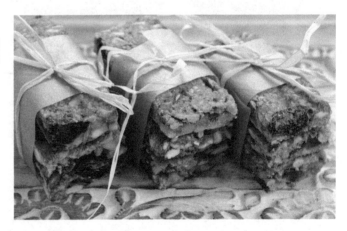

5. **Combine:** Add flax, date puree, and vanilla to dry mix; stir well.
6. **Press:** Transfer to the dish, pressing down firmly.
7. **Bake:** For 20-25 minutes until golden.
8. **Cool and Slice:** Cool before slicing into bars.

NUTRITIONAL INFORMATION (APPROXIMATE PER SERVING):

Calories: 180 | Protein: 4g | Fat: 9g | Carbs: 22g

PANCAKES & WAFFLES - A TWIST ON TRADITION

Blueberry Banana Oat Pancakes

Cooking Time: 15 minutes, Servings: 4

INGREDIENTS:

1 cup oat flour

1 banana, mashed

1 tsp baking powder

1/2 tsp cinnamon

1/4 tsp salt

1 cup almond milk

1 tbsp maple syrup (plus more for serving)

1/2 cup blueberries

Coconut oil

INSTRUCTIONS:

1. **Mix Dry:** Combine oat flour, baking powder, cinnamon, and salt.

2. **Add Wet:** Stir in banana, almond milk, and maple syrup; fold in blueberries.

3. **Cook:** Heat skillet with coconut oil, pour 1/4 cup batter per pancake. Cook until bubbles form, flip, and cook until golden.

4. **Serve:** Serve hot with maple syrup.

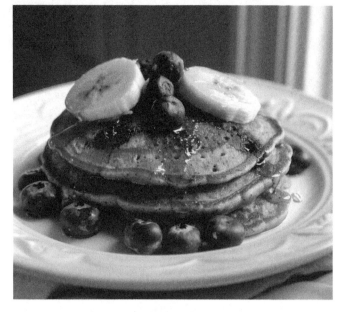

NUTRITIONAL INFORMATION (APPROXIMATE PER SERVING):

Calories: 180 | Protein: 4g | Fat: 3g | Carbs: 34g

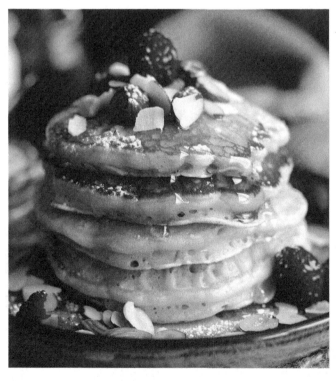

Almond and Coconut Pancakes

Cooking Time: 15 minutes, Servings: 4

INGREDIENTS:

1 cup almond flour

1/4 cup coconut flour

1 tsp baking powder

1/4 tsp salt

1 tbsp ground flaxseed + 3 tbsp water (flax egg)

1 cup coconut milk

2 tbsp melted coconut oil

1 tsp vanilla extract

Coconut shreds for garnish

INSTRUCTIONS:

1. **Mix Dry Ingredients:** In a bowl, combine almond flour, coconut flour, baking powder, and salt.

2. **Prepare Flax Egg:** Mix flaxseed with water in a small bowl; let it sit for 5 minutes until it becomes gelatinous.

3. **Add Wet Ingredients:** Mix coconut milk, melted oil, vanilla, and flax egg until combined.

4. **Pan Fry:** Heat a skillet with coconut oil. Pour 1/4 cup batter per pancake and cook for 2-3 minutes per side until golden.

5. **Serve:** Garnish with coconut shreds; serve warm with syrup or fruit.

NUTRITIONAL INFORMATION (APPROXIMATE PER SERVING):

Calories: 280 | Protein: 8g | Fat: 22g | Carbs: 15g

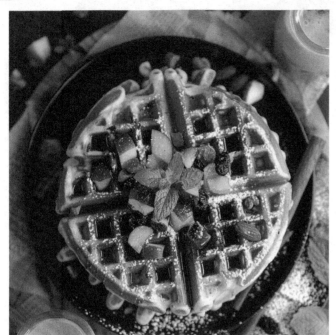

Cinnamon Apple Waffles

Cooking Time: 20 minutes, Servings: 4

INGREDIENTS:

1 cup oat flour

1 tsp baking powder

1/2 tsp cinnamon

1/4 tsp salt

1 cup almond milk

1 tbsp date puree

2 tbsp coconut oil, melted

1 medium apple, grated

INSTRUCTIONS:

1. **Mix Dry:** Combine oat flour, baking powder, cinnamon, and salt.

2. **Add Wet:** Stir in almond milk, date puree, and melted oil until smooth; fold in apple.

3. **Cook:** Preheat and grease the waffle iron. Pour batter; cook for about 5 minutes until golden.

4. **Serve:** Serve hot with date puree or toppings.

NUTRITIONAL INFORMATION
(APPROXIMATE PER SERVING):

Calories: 180 | Protein: 4g | Fat: 8g | Carbs: 25g

Pumpkin Spice Waffles

Cooking Time: 20 minutes, Servings: 4

INGREDIENTS:

1 cup buckwheat flour

1 tsp baking powder

1 tsp pumpkin spice mix

1/4 tsp salt

1 cup pumpkin puree

1 cup soy milk

2 tbsp coconut oil, melted

1 tbsp molasses

INSTRUCTIONS:

1. **Mix Dry:** Combine buckwheat flour, baking powder, pumpkin spice, and salt.

2. **Mix Wet:** In another bowl, mix pumpkin puree, soy milk, melted oil, and molasses.

3. **Combine:** Stir wet ingredients into dry until mixed.

4. **Cook:** Preheat and grease the waffle iron. Pour batter; cook for about 5 minutes until firm.

5. **Serve:** Serve warm with vegan butter or syrup.

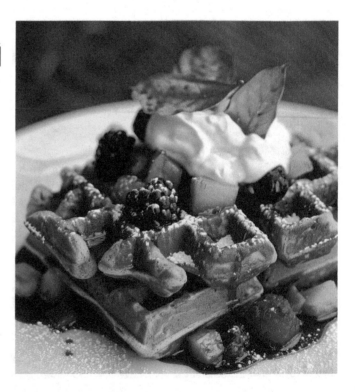

NUTRITIONAL INFORMATION
(APPROXIMATE PER SERVING):

Calories: 220 | Protein: 5g | Fat: 9g | Carbs: 32g

PUDDINGS: THE SWEET START

Creamy Avocado Chocolate Pudding

Prep Time: 10 minutes, Servings: 4

INGREDIENTS:

2 ripe avocados

1/4 cup raw cacao powder

1 tsp monk fruit sweetener (to taste)

1/2 tsp vanilla extract

Pinch of salt

1/4 cup almond milk (for consistency)

INSTRUCTIONS:

1. **Mix:** Combine all ingredients in a blender.
2. **Blend:** Blend until smooth. Adjust sweetness as needed.
3. **Chill:** Refrigerate for 30 minutes. Top with vegan whipped cream or chocolate shavings if desired.

NUTRITIONAL INFORMATION
(APPROXIMATE PER SERVING):

Calories: 230 | Protein: 3g | Fat: 15g | Carbs: 22g

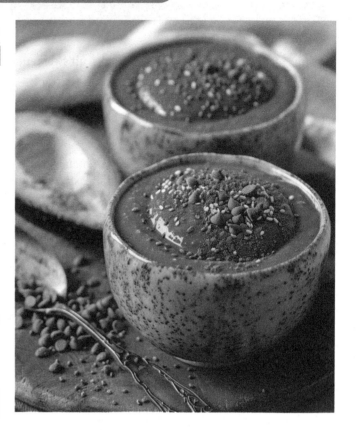

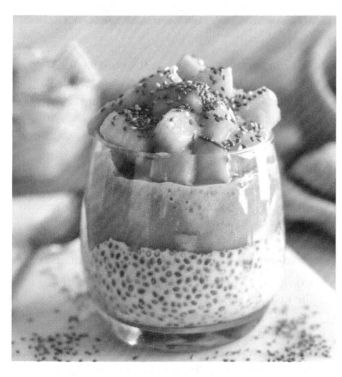

Layered Mango Chia Pudding

Prep Time: 15 minutes + chilling, Servings: 4

INGREDIENTS:

Chia Pudding:

1/3 cup chia seeds

1.5 cups coconut milk (full-fat for creamier texture)

1 tbsp maple syrup (to taste)

1 tsp vanilla extract

Mango Layer:

2 ripe mangoes, diced

1 tbsp lime juice

INSTRUCTIONS:

1. **Prepare Chia Pudding:** Mix chia seeds, coconut milk, maple syrup, and vanilla. Whisk, let sit for 5 minutes, and whisk again. Refrigerate for 4 hours or overnight.
2. **Prepare Mango Layer:** Blend mangoes and lime juice until smooth.
3. **Assemble:** Layer half of the chia pudding in four jars, then top with mango puree. Serve chilled.

NUTRITIONAL INFORMATION
(APPROXIMATE PER SERVING):

Calories: 215 | Protein: 4g | Fat: 12g | Carbs: 34g

Matcha Green Tea Pudding

Prep Time: 15 minutes (plus chilling time), Servings: 4

INGREDIENTS:

2 cups almond milk

1/4 cup chia seeds

2 tbsp matcha green tea powder

1 tsp monk fruit sweetener

1/2 tsp vanilla extract

INSTRUCTIONS:

1. **Mix Ingredients:** Mix almond milk, matcha powder, monk fruit sweetener, and vanilla extract until thoroughly combined. Stir in chia seeds.

2. **Allow to Sit:** Let the mixture sit for 5 minutes, then stir again to prevent clumping.

3. **Refrigerate:** Cover and refrigerate for at least 4 hours or overnight until the pudding has thickened and is set.

4. **Stir and Serve:** Stir well before serving. Adjust sweetness if needed. Serve chilled, topped with fresh fruit or a sprinkle of coconut flakes.

Cooking Method: No cooking. Refrigerate.

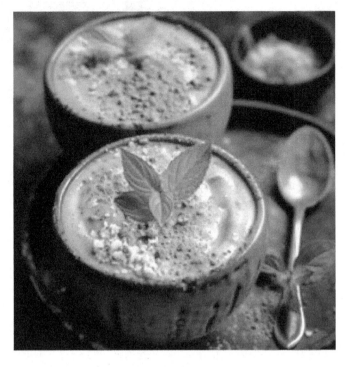

NUTRITIONAL INFORMATION (APPROX. PER SERVING):

Calories: 150 kcal | Protein: 4 g | Fat: 8 g | Carbs: 14 g

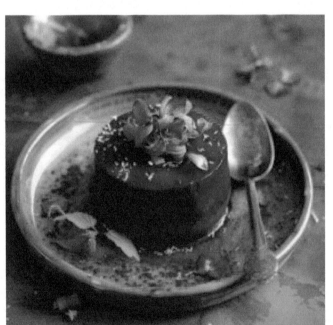

Vibrant Beetroot Coconut Pudding

Cooking Time: 15 minutes (plus chilling time), Servings: 4

INGREDIENTS:

1 medium beetroot, cooked and peeled

1 cup coconut milk

1 tsp vanilla extract

1 tbsp coconut sugar

2 tbsp arrowroot powder dissolved in 1/4 cup water

INSTRUCTIONS:

1. **Blend:** Puree the beetroot in a blender until smooth.

2. **Combine Ingredients:** Combine beetroot puree, coconut milk, vanilla extract, and coconut sugar in a saucepan. Heat over medium heat.

3. **Add Arrowroot:** Slowly add dissolved arrowroot powder to the beet mixture, stirring continuously.

4. **Cook and Serve:** Cook for about 5 minutes or until the mixture starts to thicken. Pour into serving dishes and refrigerate until set (about 2 hours). Serve chilled, garnished with a dollop of coconut cream or fresh mint.

Cooking Method: Simmering and chilling.

Arrowroot powder is an excellent alternative to cornstarch for those seeking a more natural thickening agent. It's gluten-free and creates a smooth texture without altering the flavor of the pudding. This change makes the pudding suitable for those with dietary restrictions concerning gluten and provides a cleaner label for health-conscious consumers.

NUTRITIONAL INFORMATION (APPROX. PER SERVING):

Calories: 180 kcal | Protein: 2 g | Fat: 12 g | Carbs: 16 g

Chapter 4:

LUNCHES

SAUCES AND DRESSINGS: THE FLAVOR GAME-CHANGERS

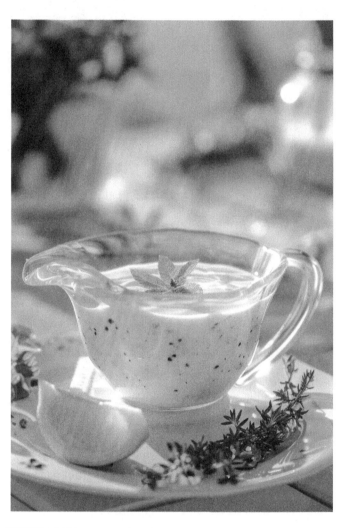

Plant-Based Caesar Dressing

Prep Time: 10 minutes, Servings: About 1 cup

INGREDIENTS:

1/2 cup soaked cashews (drained)

1/4 cup water (plus more as needed)

2 tbsp lemon juice

1 tbsp Dijon mustard

1 tbsp capers + brine

2 tsp nutritional yeast

1 garlic clove

1/2 tsp vegan Worcestershire sauce

1/2 tsp sea salt

1/4 tsp black pepper

Optional: 1 tbsp olive oil for extra richness

INSTRUCTIONS:

1. **Blend:** In a blender, mix cashews, water, lemon juice, Dijon mustard, capers, nutritional yeast, garlic, Worcestershire sauce, salt, and pepper. Blend until smooth, scraping down the sides. Add water to thin if needed.

2. **Adjust Seasoning:** Taste and adjust for tanginess or saltiness as preferred.

3. **Chill:** Refrigerate in an airtight container for 30 minutes to meld flavors and thicken slightly.

NUTRITIONAL INFORMATION (APPROXIMATE PER SERVING):

Calories: 30 kcal | Protein: 1g | Fat: 2g | Carbs: 2g

Plant-Based Oil-Free Mayo

Prep Time: 10 minutes (+ 4 hours for soaking cashews, if using), Servings: 8-10 (about 1 tbsp each)

INGREDIENTS:

1/2 cup unsweetened soy milk
(or other plant-based milk)

1 tbsp apple cider vinegar

1 tbsp lemon juice

1/2 tsp salt

1 tsp Dijon mustard

1/2 cup raw cashews, soaked for 4 hours and drained
(optional, for richness)

1-2 tbsp water (if needed, for thinning)

INSTRUCTIONS:

1. **Blend Ingredients:** In a blender, combine soy milk, vinegar, lemon juice, salt, and mustard. Blend until smooth.

2. **Add Cashews:** If using, add cashews and blend until creamy. Adjust thickness by adding water as needed.

Cooking Method: Blending.

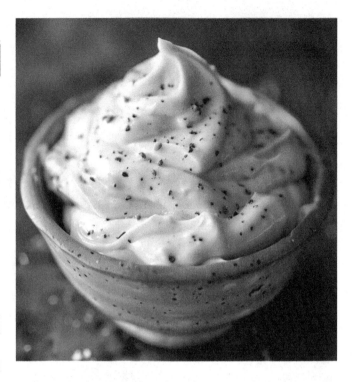

NUTRITIONAL INFORMATION
(APPROXIMATE PER SERVING):

Calories: 10-15 kcal | Protein: 0.2 g | Fat: 0.5 g | Carbs: 1 g

---

Asian-Inspired Sweet and Sour Sauce

Cooking Time: 10 minutes, Servings: 6-8 (1 tbsp each)

INGREDIENTS

1/2 cup water

1/4 cup apple cider vinegar (or white vinegar for sharper taste)

1/4 cup tamari or coconut aminos

3 tbsp maple or agave syrup

2 tbsp tomato paste

1 tbsp arrowroot powder mixed with 2 tbsp water

1 tsp sesame oil

1 clove garlic, minced

1 tsp fresh ginger, grated

1 tbsp green onions, chopped

1 tsp red chili flakes (optional)

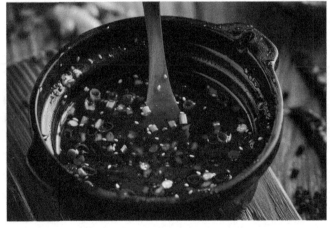

INSTRUCTIONS

1. Combine Liquid Ingredients: In a saucepan, mix water, vinegar, tamari, maple syrup, and tomato paste. Heat on medium, stirring to combine.

2. Add Flavorings: Stir in garlic, ginger, and sesame oil, then bring to a simmer.

3. Thicken: Add arrowroot mixture, stirring for 2-3 minutes until thickened.

4. Finish: Remove from heat and stir in green onions and chili flakes if using.

Cooking Method: Simmering

NUTRITIONAL INFORMATION
(APPROXIMATE PER TABLESPOON)

Calories: 25 kcal | Protein: 0.2 g | Fat: 0.5 g | Carbs: 5 g | Fiber: 0.1 g

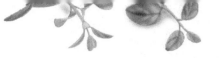

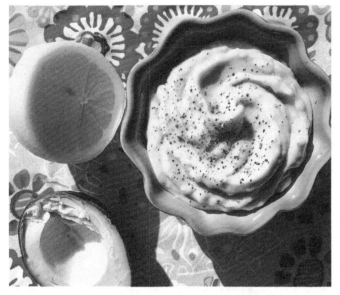

Cooking Method: Blending

NUTRITIONAL INFORMATION
(APPROXIMATE PER TABLESPOON)

Calories: 50-70 kcal | Protein: 2 g | Fat: 5 g | Carbs: 2 g

Creamy Avocado Citrus Dressing

Prep Time: 10 minutes, Servings: 6 (1 tbsp each)

INGREDIENTS

1 ripe avocado

1/4 cup fresh orange juice

1/4 cup fresh lime juice

1 clove garlic, minced

2 tbsp chopped cilantro

Salt and pepper, to taste

Optional: 1 tbsp agave syrup

Optional: Water or extra juice to thin

INSTRUCTIONS

1. **Blend:** Combine avocado, orange juice, lime juice, garlic, and cilantro in a blender until smooth.

2. **Season:** Add salt, pepper, and agave, if desired.

3. **Adjust Consistency:** Thin with water or extra citrus juice as needed.

4. **Serve:** Use immediately or refrigerate in an airtight container for up to 3 days.

Homemade Plant-Based Marinara Sauce

Prep Time: 10 minutes, Cooking Time: 30 minutes, Servings: 4 cups

INGREDIENTS

2 tbsp olive oil (optional for oil-free version)

1 large onion, finely chopped

4 cloves garlic, minced

2 cans whole peeled tomatoes (28 oz each), crushed

2 tsp dried oregano

2 tsp dried basil

1 tsp salt (to taste)

1/2 tsp black pepper

1 small carrot, grated (optional)

Pinch of red pepper flakes (optional)

INSTRUCTIONS

1. **Sauté Aromatics:** Heat olive oil (or use water/broth) in a pot over medium heat. Add onion and sauté for 5 minutes until translucent. Add garlic and sauté for another minute.

2. **Add Tomatoes:** Pour in crushed tomatoes and stir.

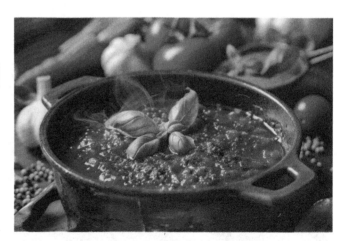

3. **Season the Sauce:** Add oregano, basil, salt, pepper, and red pepper flakes. If too acidic, add grated carrot for sweetness.

4. **Simmer:** Bring to a low boil, then reduce heat and simmer uncovered for 20-30 minutes, stirring occasionally.

NUTRITIONAL INFORMATION
(APPROXIMATE PER SERVING, 1 CUP)

Calories: 95 kcal | Protein: 2.5 g | Fat: 7 g (0 g if olive oil is omitted) | Carbs: 15.5 g

Homemade Plant-Based Ricotta

Prep Time: 4 hours 10 minutes (including soaking time), Servings: 1 cup

INGREDIENTS

1 cup raw almonds (or cashews)

1/4 cup lemon juice

1/2 cup water (plus more for soaking)

2 tbsp nutritional yeast

1 garlic clove, minced

1/2 tsp salt

Optional: Fresh herbs (basil, thyme, or parsley), finely chopped

INSTRUCTIONS

1. **Soak the Nuts:** Cover almonds with water in a bowl and soak for at least 4 hours or overnight.

2. **Prepare the Ricotta:** Drain and rinse soaked almonds. In a blender, combine almonds, lemon juice, 1/2 cup water, nutritional yeast, minced garlic, and salt. Blend until smooth and creamy. Add more water if needed for a ricotta-like consistency.

3. **Adjust Seasoning:** Taste and adjust seasoning, adding more salt or lemon juice if desired.

4. **Add Herbs (Optional):** Fold in finely chopped herbs for extra flavor.

5. **Refrigerate:** Transfer ricotta to a container and chill for at least an hour to firm up.

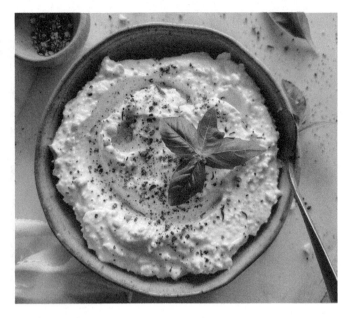

6. **Serve:** Use as a spread, filling for pasta, or topping for pizzas and salads.

Cooking Method: Soaking

NUTRITIONAL INFORMATION
(APPROXIMATE PER SERVING, 1/4 CUP)

Calories: 100 kcal | Protein: 4 g | Fat: 7 g | Carbs: 5 g | Fiber: 2 g

---

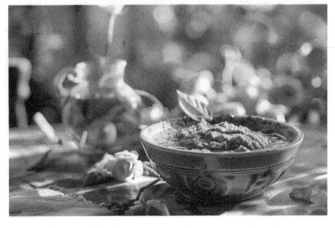

INSTRUCTIONS

1. **Blend Ingredients:** In a food processor, combine basil, nuts, and garlic. Pulse until coarsely chopped.

2. **Add Liquids:** Add nutritional yeast, lemon juice, and olive oil or water/broth. Blend until smooth, scraping down the sides as necessary. Gradually add liquid until the desired consistency is reached.

3. **Season:** Season with salt and pepper to taste.

Herbal Harmony Pesto Blend

Prep Time: 10 minutes, Servings: About 1 cup (approximately 16 tablespoons)

INGREDIENTS

2 cups fresh basil leaves

1/2 cup pine nuts or walnuts (toasted)

2-3 garlic cloves, minced

1/2 cup nutritional yeast

1/2 cup extra virgin olive oil (or water/vegetable broth for oil-free)

Juice of 1 lemon

Salt and pepper, to taste

Cooking Method: Blending

NUTRITIONAL INFORMATION
(APPROXIMATE PER TABLESPOON)

Calories: 50-70 kcal | Protein: 2 g | Fat: 5 g (less if using water or broth) | Carbs: 2 g

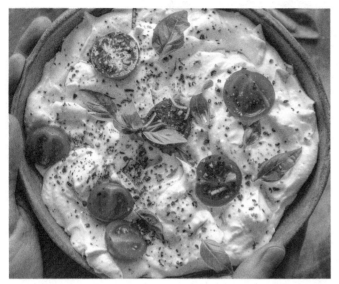

Homemade Vegan Mozzarella Cheese

Prep Time: 15 minutes,
Cooking Time: 1 hour 5 minutes (including chilling), Servings: 1 cup

INGREDIENTS

1 cup raw cashews (soaked for 4 hours, then drained)

1/3 cup water

1/4 cup refined coconut oil (melted)

1 tbsp tapioca starch

1 tbsp nutritional yeast

2 tsp lemon juice

1 tsp apple cider vinegar

1/2 tsp garlic powder

1/2 tsp salt

INSTRUCTIONS

1. **Blend Ingredients:** In a blender, combine soaked cashews, water, coconut oil, tapioca starch, nutritional yeast, lemon juice, apple cider vinegar, garlic powder, and salt. Blend until smooth.

2. **Cook the Mixture:** Transfer the mixture to a small saucepan. Heat over medium, stirring continuously for about 5 minutes until the cheese thickens and becomes stretchy.

3. **Chill:** Pour the cheese into a mold or bowl. Let it cool slightly, then refrigerate for at least 1 hour to set.

NUTRITIONAL INFORMATION
(APPROXIMATE PER SERVING)

Calories: 180 kcal | Protein: 5 g | Fat: 15 g | Carbs: 9 g | Fiber: 1 g

---

Plant-Based Parmesan Cheese

Prep Time: 5 minutes, Servings: 1 cup

INGREDIENTS

3/4 cup raw cashews (or a mix of almonds, Brazil nuts, etc.)

1/4 cup nutritional yeast

1 tsp garlic powder

1 tsp onion powder

3/4 tsp sea salt

Optional: 1/2 tsp lemon zest (for added zestiness)

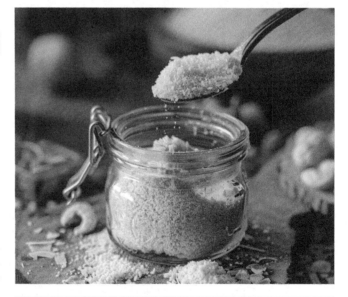

INSTRUCTIONS

1. **Blend the Ingredients:** In a food processor, combine cashews, nutritional yeast, garlic powder, onion powder, and sea salt. Pulse until you achieve a fine, grainy texture similar to grated Parmesan. Avoid over-processing into a paste; use short pulses for the best consistency.

2. **Adjust Seasonings:** Taste the mixture and adjust the seasonings as desired. Add lemon zest for extra freshness and pulse briefly to combine.

3. **Serve:** Sprinkle over pizzas, pasta, risotto, salads, or any dish where traditional Parmesan cheese is desired.

Cooking Method: Blending.

NUTRITIONAL INFORMATION
(APPROXIMATE PER TABLESPOON)

Calories: 30 kcal | Protein: 2 g | Fat: 2 g | Carbs: 2 g | Fiber: 1 g

Caesar Salad with Tempeh and Avocado

Cooking Time: 30 minutes, Servings: 4

INGREDIENTS

For the Salad:

200 g (about 7 ounces) tempeh, diced

1 large ripe avocado, sliced

1 head romaine lettuce, chopped

1 cup cherry tomatoes, halved

Plant-Based Caesar Dressing Chapter 4

INSTRUCTIONS

1. **Prepare the Tempeh:** Sauté the tempeh cubes in a skillet over medium heat until golden brown. Set aside to cool.

2. **Make the Dressing:** Plant-Based Caesar Dressing Chapter 4

3. **Assemble the Salad:** In a large salad bowl, combine chopped romaine lettuce, sliced avocado, cherry

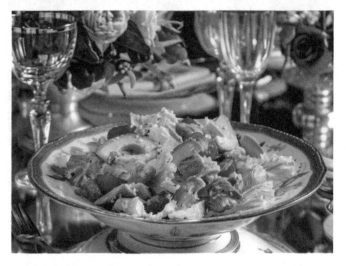

tomatoes, and cooled tempeh. Drizzle with Caesar dressing and toss well to coat.

NUTRITIONAL INFORMATION (PER SERVING)

Calories: 250 kcal | Protein: 12 g | Fat: 15 g | Carbs: 18 g | Fiber: 6 g | Sugars: 5 g | Cholesterol: 0 mg | Sodium: 200 mg

---

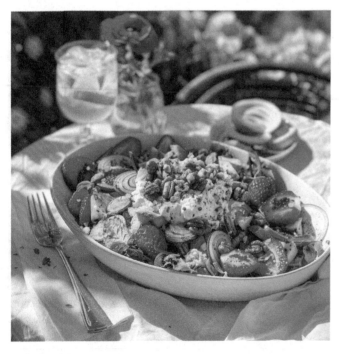

Strawberry Salad with Avocado and Homemade Ricotta

Prep Time: 20 minutes, Servings: 4

INGREDIENTS

2 cups fresh strawberries, sliced

1 large avocado, diced

1/4 cup red onion, thinly sliced

1/2 cup homemade plant-based ricotta

1/4 cup toasted pecans

4 cups fresh baby spinach or mixed greens

For the Dressing: Homemade Plant-Based Ricotta. Chapter 4

INSTRUCTIONS

1. **Prepare the Dressing:** Homemade Plant-Based Ricotta. Chapter 4

2. **Assemble the Salad:** In a large bowl, combine strawberries, avocado, red onion, and greens. Add dollops of ricotta and sprinkle with pecans.

3. **Dress and Serve:** Drizzle dressing over the salad just before serving. Cooking Method: No cooking. Blending.

NUTRITIONAL INFORMATION
(APPROXIMATE PER SERVING)

Calories: 250 kcal | Protein: 6 g | Fat: 18 g | Carbs: 19 g | Fiber: 5 g

OH, MY BOWL: THE ULTIMATE BOWL GUIDE

Bowls - the culinary rock stars of the modern, health-conscious foodie scene. Each bowl is a masterpiece screaming to be captured in a photo, boasting uniqueness. And the cherry on top? The convenience of grab-and-go. Picture this: you unveil your bowl at lunch among colleagues, and boom – it's an instant 'wow' moment.

Start with your favorite bowl. Now, let's get wildly creative – fill it with a kaleidoscope of flavors and a rainbow of colors. Dive into each category, picking one, two, or a whole medley of ingredients. Follow the list step by step. Missing something? No problem. Choose your ingredients based on what's available to you.

Start with the Base: Choosing your base is like laying the foundation of a house. Options like rice, buckwheat, and quinoa each add their unique texture and nutrients. Experiment away! Quinoa today, amaranth tomorrow.

Protein—Your Powerhouse: Beans, chickpeas, and tofu aren't just sources of protein; they're your all-day energy. Try marinated tofu or spicy chickpeas to see how they impact your overall well-being and vitality.

Ingredient Play: This is where the real magic happens. Add red onion for sharpness, pineapple for sweetness, or wakame for a sea-flavored twist.

The Topping Transformation: Just when you thought your bowl couldn't get any better, enter the game-changing toppings. A sprinkle of chia seeds, a dash of sesame, or a handful of dried fruits are not just toppings – they transform your bowl, adding delightful textures and flavors.

Sauce—The Wizard of Your Dish: Sauce can transform your bowl. Experiment with various types, from spicy ginger to creamy peanut butter, to find the one that awakens your taste buds.

Embark on a Spice Odyssey: Each spice is a gateway to new flavor realms. Turmeric for a vibrant hue and hint of earthy mystery, cumin for that warm, aromatic embrace, and paprika for a sweet, spicy whirlwind.

Every bowl is an opportunity to discover something new. Don't be afraid to experiment. Change one ingredient, and you'll have a completely different experience. Remember, there are no rules – just your taste, choice, and creativity. Create, experiment, and enjoy each unique bowl!

Create Your Unique POKE BOWL!

Regular bowl: 1 base and add 4 ingredients, 1 protein, 1 topping, and 1 sauce.
Grand bowl: 1 base, 5 ingredients, 1 protein, 2 toppings, and 1 sauce.

BASE:

- Rice
- Buckwheat
- Green Lentils
- Quinoa
- Bulgur*
- Amaranth
- Various Pasta (Whole Wheat*, Spelt*, Gluten-free options)
- Rice Noodles
- Soba Noodles (Buckwheat)
- Udon Noodles*
- Couscous*
- Orzo*
- Quinoa Pasta
- Zucchini Noodles (Zoodles)
- Shirataki Noodles (Konjac Yam)
- Vegan Ramen Noodles*

INGREDIENTS:

- Salad, Kale, Cooked, Pak-Choi, Spinach etc
- Cucumber
- Edamame
- Red Cabbage
- Radish
- Carrot
- Tomato
- Chioggia Beetroot
- Red Onion
- Celery
- Fermented Vegetables
- Microgreens Seeds
- Apple
- Pineapple
- Pomegranate
- Corn
- Mango
- Fresh Berries (Strawberries, Blueberries, Raspberries, Blackberries, etc.)
- Wakame
- Vegan Cream Cheese
- Ingredient of the Moment

PROTEIN:

- Hummus
- Falafel*
- Marine Tofu (Thai style) / Grilled Tofu
- Assorted Vegan Proteins (check recipes)
- Hulled Hemp Seeds (Hemp Hearts)
- Beans (Black Beans, Kidney Beans, Pinto Beans, etc.)
- Chickpeas (Garbanzo Beans)

TOPPINGS:

- Cilantro
- Shallot
- Sesame Seeds
- Sea Ginger
- Fried Onions*
- Pumpkin Seeds
- Peanuts
- Jalapeños

- **Nuts:** Almonds, Brazil Nuts, Cashews, Hazelnuts, Macadamias, Pecans, Pine Nuts, Pistachios, Walnuts, Peanuts
- **Seeds:** Pumpkin, Flax, Sesame, Poppy, Sunflower, Psyllium, Chia

- **Dried Fruits:** (dates, apricots, raisins, dried cranberries, figs, etc.)
- Nutritional Yeast Flakes

EXTRAS:

- Avocado
- Mango
- Wakame
- Ginger
- Lime

- Lemon
- Vegan Cream Cheese
- Double Base, Ingredient, Topping, Protein, or Sauce

SAUCES: (ASSORTMENT, CHECK SAUCE RECIPES):

- Vinegar
- Guacamole
- Mayo (vegan if for plant-based diet)

- Peanut Butter
- Spicy Ginger

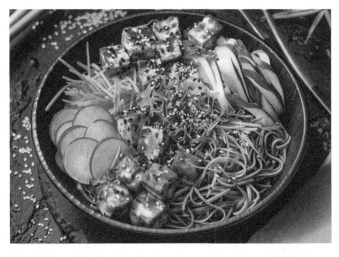

Zen Garden Poke Bowl Recipe

Cooking Time: 30 minutes, Servings: 2

INGREDIENTS

1 cup cooked pak choi, roughly chopped

1 large radish, thinly sliced

1 carrot, julienned

1/4 cup microgreens

Base:
200 g soba noodles

Protein:
200 g marine tofu (marinated tofu with seaweed flavor)

Topping:
1 tbsp sea ginger (pickled ginger); 2 tbsp pumpkin seeds

Sauce:
1/2 ripe avocado; Juice of 1 orange; Juice of 1 lime, 1 clove garlic, minced; 1/4 cup cilantro, chopped; Salt and pepper to taste

INSTRUCTIONS

1. **Cook Soba Noodles:** Boil water, add noodles, and cook 4-5 minutes. Drain and rinse under cold water.

2. **Prepare the Sauce:** Blend avocado, orange juice, lime juice, garlic, and cilantro until smooth. Season with salt and pepper; add water for desired consistency if needed.

3. **Prepare the Tofu:** If not pre-marinated, marinate tofu in soy sauce, lime juice, and seaweed flakes for 10-15 minutes. Grill or pan-fry until golden brown.

4. **Assemble the Bowl:** Place soba noodles in each bowl. Top with pak choi, radish, carrots, and microgreens. Add tofu, sprinkle with sea ginger and pumpkin seeds, and drizzle with sauce.

NUTRITIONAL INFORMATION
(APPROXIMATE PER SERVING)

Calories: 550 kcal | Protein: 25 g | Fat: 20 g | Carbs: 65 g | Fiber: 10 g

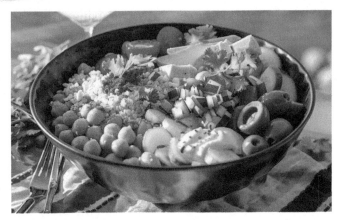

Mediterranean Chickpea Poke Bowl Recipe

Cooking Time: 30 minutes, Servings: 2

INGREDIENTS

1 large tomato, diced

2 cups fresh spinach, roughly chopped

1 small red onion, thinly sliced

1/2 cup kalamata olives, pitted and sliced

1 cucumber, diced

Base: 1 cup bulgur

Protein: 1 cup cooked chickpeas

Topping: 2 tbsp nutritional yeast flakes, 1 avocado, diced

Sauce: 1/2 cup vegan cream cheese, Juice of 1 lemon, 1 tbsp chopped fresh herbs (parsley and dill)

INSTRUCTIONS

1. **Prepare the Bulgur:** Rinse bulgur. In a saucepan, bring 2 cups of water to boil. Add bulgur, reduce heat to low, cover, and simmer for 10-15 minutes until water is absorbed. Fluff with a fork and let cool slightly.

2. **Make the Sauce:** In a bowl, blend vegan cream cheese with lemon juice and fresh herbs until smooth.

3. **Assemble the Bowl:** Divide bulgur into bowls. Top with diced tomato, chopped spinach, sliced onion, olives, cucumber, and chickpeas. Sprinkle with nutritional yeast and diced avocado. Drizzle with sauce

NUTRITIONAL INFORMATION
(APPROXIMATE PER SERVING)

Calories: 560 kcal | Protein: 19 g | Fat: 20 g | Carbs: 80 g | Fiber: 19 g | Sugar: 8 g

---

Tropical Tofu Poke Bowl

Cooking Time: 30 minutes, Servings: 2

INGREDIENTS

1 mango, peeled and diced

1 cucumber, julienned

1 cup edamame, shelled and cooked

1 cup red cabbage, shredded

Base: 1 cup quinoa

Protein: 200 g tofu, pressed and grilled

Topping: 1 tbsp sesame seeds; A handful of cilantro, chopped

Sauce: 2 tbsp soy sauce; 1 tbsp grated ginger; 1 tbsp rice vinegar; 1 tsp sesame oil; 1 tsp chili flakes (adjust to taste); 1 tbsp date puree (as a natural sweetener)

INSTRUCTIONS

1. **Prepare the Quinoa:** Rinse quinoa. In a saucepan, bring 2 cups of water to a boil. Add quinoa, reduce heat to low, cover, and simmer for 15 minutes. Remove from heat, let stand for 5 minutes, then fluff with a fork.

2. **Grill the Tofu:** Slice tofu into 1/2-inch thick pieces. Lightly oil a grill pan over medium heat. Grill tofu for 3-4 minutes on each side until charred and heated through.

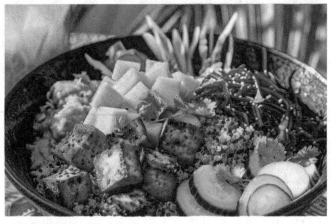

3. **Make the Sauce:** In a small bowl, mix soy sauce, grated ginger, rice vinegar, sesame oil, chili flakes, and date puree until smooth.

4. **Assemble the Bowl:** Divide quinoa into bowls. Top with diced mango, julienned cucumber, cooked edamame, and shredded cabbage. Place grilled tofu on top. Sprinkle with sesame seeds and chopped cilantro. Drizzle with sauce before serving.

NUTRITIONAL INFORMATION
(APPROXIMATE PER SERVING)

Calories: 560 kcal | Protein: 26 g | Fat: 18 g | Carbs: 74 g | Fiber: 10 g | Sugar: 18 g

Herbal Lentil & Hummus Delight

Cooking Time: 30 minutes, Servings: 2

INGREDIENTS

1 cucumber, sliced

1 cup cherry tomatoes, halved

1/2 red onion, thinly sliced

1/2 cup kalamata olives, pitted and halved

Base: 2 cups mixed salad greens

Protein: 1 cup lentils; 1/2 tsp cumin; 1/2 tsp coriander; 1/2 tsp smoked paprika

Topping: 1/2 cup homemade plant-based ricotta (from blended almonds or cashews); 1 avocado, diced

Sauce: 1 cup hummus; 2 tbsp olive oil; juice of 1 lemon; water as needed

NUTRITIONAL INFORMATION (APPROX. PER SERVING)

Calories: 560 | Protein: 20 g | Fat: 25 g | Carbs: 65 g | Fiber: 18 g | Sugar: 8 g

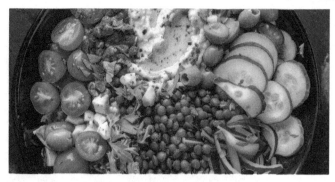

INSTRUCTIONS

1. **Cook Lentils:** Rinse lentils. In a pot, cover with water, bring to boil, then simmer with spices for 20-25 minutes until tender. Drain and cool.

2. **Prepare Hummus Sauce:** Blend hummus, olive oil, and lemon juice. Add water for consistency.

3. **Make Ricotta:** Blend soaked almonds/cashews with lemon juice, nutritional yeast, and salt until creamy.

4. **Assemble Bowl:** Layer greens, then top with lentils, cucumber, tomatoes, onion, olives, ricotta, and avocado. Drizzle with sauce.

4. SOUPS AND STEWS: THE HEARTWARMING STAPLES

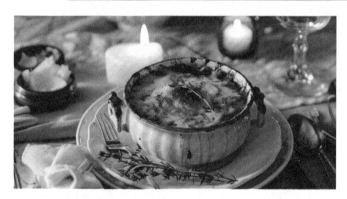

INSTRUCTIONS

1. **Caramelize the Onions:** In a large pot, add a small amount of vegetable broth over medium heat. Sauté onions, adding date puree as they soften. Cook, stirring frequently, until caramelized (about 30-40 minutes), adding water or broth as needed to prevent burning.

2. **Add Flavorings and Cook the Soup:** Stir in balsamic vinegar, thyme, and bay leaf. Cook for 1-2 minutes. Pour in vegetable broth, bring to a boil, then reduce heat and simmer for 20 minutes.

3. **Prepare Bread and Cheese Topping:** Toast the bread until crispy. Ladle soup into oven-safe bowls, top with toasted bread, and sprinkle with grated mozzarella.Chapter 4

4. **Broil:** Preheat the oven's broiler. Broil the soup until cheese melts and turns golden brown (3-5 minutes).

Plant-Based French Onion Soup with Date Puree

Cooking Time: 1 hour, Servings: 4

INGREDIENTS

4 large onions, thinly sliced

1-2 tbsp date puree (to taste)

1 tbsp balsamic vinegar

6 cups vegetable broth

1 tsp dried thyme

1 bay leaf

Salt and black pepper (Himalayan salt or celery salt preferred)

4 slices plant-based bread or flatbreads for serving

1 cup grated plant-based mozzarella cheese Chapter 4

5. **Serve:** Enjoy hot, garnished with additional herbs or pepper if desired.

Cooking Method: Caramelize, simmer, and broil.

NUTRITIONAL INFORMATION (APPROX. PER SERVING)

Calories: 280-320 kcal | Protein: 10-12 g | Fat: 7-9 g | Carbs: 45-50 g | Fiber: 6-8 g | Sugars: 14-18 g | Sodium: 800-1000 mg (varies by broth and cheese used)

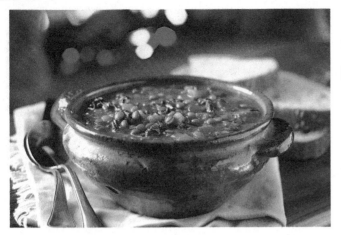

Spicy Lentil and Spinach Soup

Prep Time: 10 min, Cooking Time: 30 min, Servings: 4

INGREDIENTS

- 1-2 tbsp vegetable broth (or water) for sautéing
- 1 large onion, chopped
- 2 carrots, diced
- 2 celery stalks, diced
- 2 cloves garlic, minced
- 1 tsp ground cumin
- 1 tsp chili powder
- 1/2 tsp smoked paprika
- 1 cup red lentils, rinsed and drained
- 4 cups vegetable broth
- 2 cups water
- 2 cups fresh spinach, roughly chopped
- Himalayan salt or celery salt, to taste
- Juice of half a lemon (optional)

INSTRUCTIONS

1. **Sauté Vegetables:** In a large pot, heat 1-2 tablespoons of vegetable broth or water over medium heat. Add onion, carrots, and celery; cook for about 5 minutes until softened. Stir in garlic, cumin, chili powder, and smoked paprika; cook for 1 minute until fragrant.

2. **Cook Lentils:** Add red lentils, vegetable broth, and water. Bring to a boil, then reduce heat to a simmer. Cover and simmer for about 20 minutes, until lentils are tender.

3. **Add Spinach:** Stir in chopped spinach and simmer for another 5 minutes until wilted.

4. **Season and Serve:** Season with Himalayan or celery salt to taste. For extra zest, stir in lemon juice. Serve hot with crusty bread or a side salad.

Cooking Method: Sauté and simmer.

NUTRITIONAL INFORMATION (APPROX. PER SERVING)

Calories: 260 kcal | Protein: 18 g | Fat: 4 g | Carbs: 42 g | Fiber: 15 g | Sugar: 6 g

---

Butternut Squash and Ginger Soup: A Healthy Delight

Cooking Time: 30 minutes, Servings: 4

INGREDIENTS

Vegetable broth or water for sautéing

1 onion, chopped

2 tbsp fresh ginger, minced

1 butternut squash, peeled and cubed

4 cups vegetable broth

Himalayan salt or celery salt, to taste

Optional: Coconut milk for drizzling

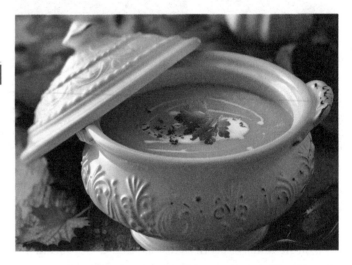

INSTRUCTIONS

1. **Sauté Aromatics:** In a large pot, heat a splash of vegetable broth or water over medium heat. Add onion and ginger; sauté until the onion is translucent, adding more broth if needed to prevent sticking.

2. **Cook the Squash:** Add cubed butternut squash and 4 cups of vegetable broth. Bring to a boil, then reduce heat and simmer for about 25 minutes, until the squash is tender.

3. **Blend the Soup:** Use an immersion blender directly in the pot or transfer to a blender. Blend until smooth and creamy, then return to the pot if needed.

4. **Season and Serve:** Season with Himalayan or celery salt. Drizzle with coconut milk if desired, and serve hot.

NUTRITIONAL INFORMATION (APPROX. PER SERVING)

Calories: 150 kcal | Protein: 2 g | Fat: 1 g (without coconut milk) | Carbs: 35 g | Fiber: 6 g | Sugar: 7 g

Wild Mushroom and Barley Soup Recipe

Cooking Time: 50 minutes, Servings: 4

INGREDIENTS

Vegetable broth or water for sautéing

1 large onion, finely chopped

2 cloves garlic, minced

450 g assorted wild mushrooms (e.g., porcini, shiitake, chanterelle), roughly chopped

3/4 cup pearl barley, rinsed

6 cups vegetable broth

2 tbsp fresh thyme, chopped

1 bay leaf

Himalayan salt or celery salt, to taste

Freshly ground black pepper, to taste

INSTRUCTIONS

1. **Sauté Aromatics:** In a large pot, heat a splash of vegetable broth or water over medium heat. Add onion and garlic; sauté until the onion is translucent. Add more broth as needed to prevent sticking.

2. **Add Mushrooms:** Stir in the wild mushrooms and cook for about 10 minutes, until softened and juices are released.

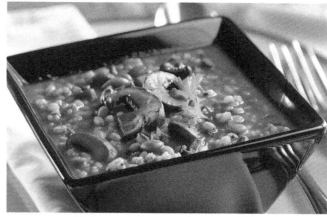

3. **Cook Barley:** Add pearl barley, 6 cups of vegetable broth, thyme, and bay leaf. Bring to a boil, then reduce to a simmer. Cover and let simmer for 30-35 minutes, until barley is tender.

4. **Season and Serve:** Remove the bay leaf. Season with Himalayan or celery salt and black pepper to taste. Serve hot, ideally in a deep black square bowl for a rustic presentation.

NUTRITIONAL INFORMATION (APPROX. PER SERVING)

Calories: 250 kcal | Protein: 8 g | Fat: 1 g | Carbs: 52 g | Fiber: 10 g

---

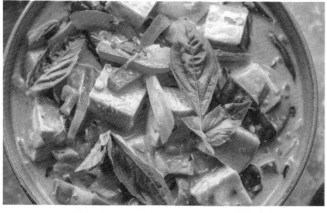

Thai Coconut Curry with Tofu

Cooking Time: 30 minutes, Servings: 4

INGREDIENTS

400 g firm tofu, pressed and cubed

1 tbsp coconut oil (or water for an oil-free version)

1 red bell pepper, thinly sliced

1 green bell pepper, thinly sliced

1 medium onion, thinly sliced

2 cloves garlic, minced

1 tbsp fresh ginger, grated

2 tbsp Thai red curry paste (ensure vegan)

1 can (14 oz) coconut milk

1 cup vegetable broth

1 tbsp soy sauce or tamari

1 tbsp maple syrup

Juice of 1 lime

1/2 cup bamboo shoots

1/2 cup fresh basil leaves

Himalayan salt, to taste

INSTRUCTIONS

1. **Prepare Tofu:** Heat coconut oil in a large skillet over medium heat. Add tofu and fry for 8-10 minutes until golden brown. Remove and set aside.

2. **Sauté Vegetables:** In the same skillet, add more coconut oil or a splash of water. Add onion, garlic, and ginger; sauté until onion is translucent. Add bell peppers and cook until just tender.

3. **Make the Curry:** Stir in curry paste and cook for 1 minute until fragrant. Add coconut milk, vegetable broth, soy sauce, and maple syrup; bring to a simmer. Return tofu and add bamboo shoots. Let simmer for about 10 minutes until slightly thickened.

4. **Final Touches:** Stir in lime juice and basil. Season with Himalayan salt to taste.

5. **Serving:** Serve hot over steamed rice or with flatbread. Garnish with additional basil if desired.

NUTRITIONAL INFORMATION (APPROX.PER SERVING)

Calories: 350 kcal | Protein: 12 g | Fat: 25 g | Carbs: 18 g

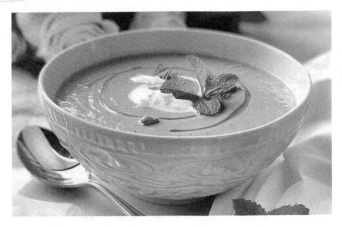

Green Pea and Mint Soup

Cooking Time: 25 minutes, Servings: 4

INGREDIENTS

1 tbsp vegetable broth (for sautéing)

1 medium onion, finely chopped

2 cloves garlic, minced

4 cups fresh or frozen green peas

4 cups vegetable broth

1/4 cup fresh mint leaves, plus extra for garnish

Salt and black pepper to taste

Optional garnishes: coconut cream, lemon zest, crushed pistachios

INSTRUCTIONS

1. **Sauté Onion and Garlic:** In a large pot, heat vegetable broth over medium heat. Add chopped onion and sauté until translucent. Add garlic and cook for another minute until fragrant.

2. **Cook the Peas:** Add green peas and vegetable broth to the pot. Bring to a boil, then reduce heat and simmer for about 10 minutes, or until peas are tender.

3. **Add Mint and Blend:** Stir in fresh mint leaves. Remove from heat and use an immersion blender to puree until smooth. Alternatively, blend in batches in a regular blender and return to the pot.

4. **Season and Serve:** Reheat gently if needed. Season with salt and black pepper to taste. Serve hot or chilled, garnished with extra mint, a drizzle of coconut cream, lemon zest, or crushed pistachios.

NUTRITIONAL INFORMATION (APPROX. PER SERVING)

Calories: 180 kcal | Protein: 12 g | Fat: 1 g | Carbs: 34 g | Fiber: 12 g | Sugar: 15 g

---

Thick Jackfruit Stew

Cooking Time: 1 hour 20 minutes, Servings: 4

INGREDIENTS

500 g jackfruit pulp (fresh or canned), seeded and chopped

2 medium carrots, diced

2 celery stalks, diced

1 large onion, finely chopped

2 cloves garlic, minced

2 tbsp tomato paste

1 tbsp smoked paprika

1 tsp ground coriander

1/2 tsp chili powder

400 g chopped tomatoes in their juice

400 ml vegetable broth

2 bay leaves

Himalayan salt or celery salt, to taste

Freshly ground black pepper, to taste

Fresh herbs for garnish (e.g., parsley or cilantro)

INSTRUCTIONS

1. **Prepare Jackfruit:** If using canned jackfruit, rinse and squeeze to remove excess liquid.

2. **Sauté Aromatics:** Heat vegetable broth in a large saucepan over medium heat. Add onion and garlic; cook until onion softens (about 5 minutes). Add carrots and celery; fry for another 5 minutes.

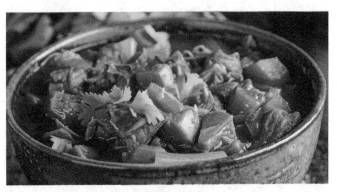

3. **Add Jackfruit and Spices:** Stir in jackfruit, tomato paste, smoked paprika, coriander, and chili powder. Mix well and fry for 5 minutes.

4. **Add Liquids and Simmer:** Add chopped tomatoes, vegetable broth, and bay leaves. Bring to a boil, then reduce heat, cover, and simmer for 40-50 minutes, stirring occasionally until thickened.

5. **Season and Serve:** Season with salt and pepper to taste. Let sit, covered, for 10 minutes before serving. Garnish with fresh herbs.

NUTRITIONAL INFORMATION (APPROX. PER SERVING)

Calories: 220 kcal | Protein: 4 g | Fat: 1 g | Carbs: 50 g | Fiber: 8 g

Plant Goulash Based on Mushrooms and Lentils

Cooking Time: 1 hour 15 minutes, Servings: 4

INGREDIENTS

300 g champignons, cut into large pieces

200 g red lentils, pre-cooked until half cooked

2 large carrots, diced

2 celery stalks, diced

1 large onion, finely chopped

2 cloves garlic, minced

1 tbsp paprika

1 tsp ground cumin

1/2 tsp ground black pepper

400 g chopped tomatoes in their juice

500 ml vegetable broth

2 bay leaves

2 tbsp tomato paste

Himalayan salt or celery salt, to taste

Fresh herbs for garnish (e.g., parsley)

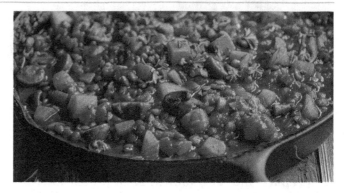

INSTRUCTIONS

1. **Sauté Aromatics:** Heat vegetable broth in a large saucepan over medium heat. Add onion and garlic; sauté until translucent (about 5 minutes).

2. **Add Vegetables:** Stir in carrots and celery; cook for another 5 minutes until softened. Add mushrooms, paprika, cumin, and black pepper; stir-fry for 5 minutes.

3. **Add Liquids:** Mix in chopped tomatoes, tomato paste, bay leaves, and vegetable broth. Bring to a boil.

4. **Simmer:** Reduce heat, add pre-cooked lentils, and cover. Simmer over low heat for 40 minutes, stirring occasionally until thickened.

5. **Season and Serve:** Season with salt to taste. Remove from heat and let sit, covered, for 10 minutes before serving. Garnish with fresh herbs.

NUTRITIONAL INFORMATION (APPROX. PER SERVING)

Calories: 250 kcal | Protein: 14 g | Fat: 3 g | Carbs: 45 g | Fiber: 12 g

---

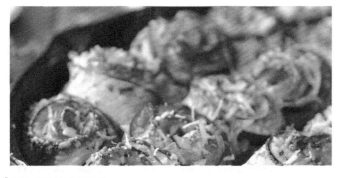

INSTRUCTIONS

1. **Prepare Zucchini:** Preheat oven to 375°F (190°C). Season zucchini slices with salt and pepper. Grill for 1-2 minutes on each side until tender. Set aside.

2. **Make Filling:** Sauté onion and garlic until translucent. Add mushrooms and cook until golden. Stir in pine nuts, basil, parsley, and nutritional yeast (if using). Season with salt and pepper.

3. **Prepare Tomato Sauce:** In a saucepan, combine crushed tomatoes, garlic, oregano, salt, and pepper. Simmer for 10 minutes.

4. **Assemble Rolls:** Place a spoonful of filling on each zucchini slice, roll tightly, and place seam-side down in a baking dish.

5. **Add Topping:** Sprinkle mozzarella over the zucchini rolls and pour the tomato sauce on top.

6. **Bake:** Bake for 15-20 minutes until the cheese melts.

Zucchini Rolls with Herbed Mushroom and Pine Nut Stuffing

Prep Time: 45 min, Cooking Time: 20 min, Servings: 4

INGREDIENTS

For the Zucchini Rolls:

4 zucchinis, sliced lengthwise; Salt and pepper to taste

For the Filling:

1 onion, finely chopped; 2 garlic cloves, minced; 1 cup mushrooms, chopped; 1/4 cup pine nuts; 1/4 cup fresh basil, chopped; 1/4 cup fresh parsley, chopped; 1 tbsp nutritional yeast (optional); Salt and pepper to taste

For the Tomato Sauce:

2 cups crushed tomatoes; 1 garlic clove, minced; 1 tsp dried oregano; Salt and pepper to taste

Topping:

1/2 cup shredded plant-based mozzarella

NUTRITIONAL INFORMATION (APPROX. PER SERVING)

Calories: 250 kcal | Protein: 8 g | Fat: 15 g | Carbs: 22 g | Fiber: 5 g

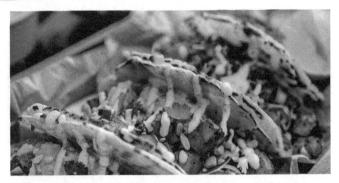

Vegan Charred Sweet Potato and Bell Pepper Tacos with Avocado Lime Sauce

Prep Time: 35 min, Cooking Time: 25 min, Servings: 4

INGREDIENTS

For the Tacos

8 Chickpea or Grain-Free Taco Tortillas; 2 large sweet potatoes, peeled and diced; 2 large bell peppers (1 red, 1 yellow), sliced; 1 teaspoon smoked paprika; 1 teaspoon ground cumin; Salt and pepper to taste; Fresh cilantro, for garnish; Toasted pine nuts, for garnish

For the Avocado Lime Sauce

1 ripe avocado; Juice of 1 lime; 1/4 cup cilantro, chopped; 1 clove garlic; 2 tablespoons vegan yogurt or soaked cashews; Salt and pepper to taste; Water, as needed

NUTRITIONAL INFORMATION (APPROX. PER SERVING)

Calories: 360 kcal | Protein: 9 g | Fat: 19 g | Carbs: 45 g | Fiber: 10 g

INSTRUCTIONS

1. **Prepare the Vegetables:** Preheat oven to 400°F (200°C). Spread diced sweet potatoes and sliced bell peppers on a parchment-lined baking sheet. Season with smoked paprika, cumin, salt, and pepper. Roast for 20-25 minutes until tender and charred.

2. **Make the Avocado Lime Sauce:** Blend avocado, lime juice, cilantro, garlic, and yogurt or cashews until smooth. Season with salt and pepper. Add water for a creamy consistency.

3. **Assemble the Tacos:** Warm tortillas in a skillet until pliable. Fill with roasted vegetables, drizzle with avocado lime sauce, and garnish with cilantro and pine nuts.

Thai Vegetable Cutlets with Coconut-Ginger Sauce

Cooking Time: 45 minutes, Servings: 4

INGREDIENTS

For the Cutlets

1 cup cooked chickpeas, mashed; 1 cup red cabbage, finely shredded; 1/2 cup grated carrots; 1/4 cup fresh cilantro, chopped; 2 tablespoons fresh ginger, minced; 1 garlic clove, minced; Zest and juice of 1 lime; 1 tablespoon tamari or soy sauce; 1/2 cup coconut flakes; Himalayan or celery salt, to taste; 2 tablespoons coconut oil, for frying

For the Coconut-Ginger Sauce

1 can (14 oz) coconut milk; 2 tablespoons grated ginger; 1 tablespoon soy sauce; 1 tablespoon maple or agave syrup; Juice of 1 lime; Salt, to taste; Optional: Red chili flakes for heat

INSTRUCTIONS

1. **Prepare the Cutlet Mixture:** In a bowl, combine mashed chickpeas, cabbage, carrots, cilantro, ginger, garlic, lime zest, lime juice, tamari (or soy sauce), and coconut flakes. Season with salt to taste.

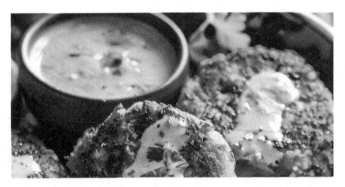

2. **Form the Cutlets:** Divide the mixture into equal portions and shape each into a half-inch thick patty.

3. **Cook the Cutlets:** Heat coconut oil in a skillet over medium heat. Fry the cutlets for 4-5 minutes on each side until golden brown and crispy. Drain on paper towels.

4. **Prepare the Coconut-Ginger Sauce:** In a saucepan, mix coconut milk, ginger, soy sauce, maple syrup, and lime juice. Simmer over medium heat, stirring frequently. Season with salt and optional chili flakes, and let thicken for 5-7 minutes.

NUTRITIONAL INFORMATION (APPROX. PER SERVING)

Calories: 300 kcal | Protein: 8 g | Fat: 18 g | Carbs: 28 g | Fiber: 6 g

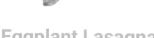

Eggplant Lasagna

Prep Time: 30 min, Cook Time: 45 min, Servings: 6

INGREDIENTS

Lasagna

2 large eggplants, sliced lengthwise (1/4-inch thick)

Salt and pepper, to taste

3 cups marinara sauce

2 cups vegan mozzarella, shredded

1 cup vegan parmesan, grated

Ricotta Filling

1 (14 oz) block firm tofu, crumbled

1/4 cup nutritional yeast

2 tbsp lemon juice

1 garlic clove, minced

1/2 cup fresh basil, chopped

Salt and pepper, to taste

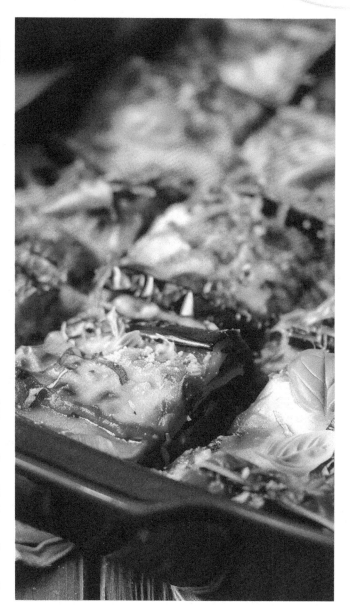

INSTRUCTIONS

1. **Prepare Eggplant:** Preheat oven to 375°F (190°C). Season eggplant with salt and pepper; roast on a lined baking sheet for 20-25 minutes until tender.

2. **Make Filling:** Mix tofu, nutritional yeast, lemon juice, garlic, basil, salt, and pepper until resembling ricotta.

3. **Assemble:** In a baking dish, layer marinara, roasted eggplant, ricotta, mozzarella, and parmesan. Repeat layers, finishing with marinara and cheese.

4. **Bake:** Cover with foil; bake for 25 minutes. Remove foil and bake 10-15 more minutes until golden.

5. **Serve:** Cool for 10 minutes before slicing. Garnish with basil or parsley if desired.

NUTRITIONAL INFORMATION (APPROX. PER SERVING)

Calories: 320 kcal | Protein: 15 g | Fat: 18 g | Carbs: 25 g | Fiber: 8 g

Chapter 5:

DINNERS

MAIN COURSES: REDEFINING THE PLANT-BASED FEAST

Plant-Based Spiral Vegetable Tart with Sweet Potato

Cooking Time: 1 hour 30 minutes, Servings: 6-8

INGREDIENTS

For the Crust
- 1 1/2 cups almond or oat flour
- 1/4 cup olive or melted coconut oil
- 1/4 cup cold water
- 1/2 tsp salt

For the Filling
- 1 cup hummus
- 1 medium sweet potato, thinly sliced
- 1 zucchini, thinly sliced
- 1 carrot, thinly sliced
- 1 eggplant, thinly sliced
- 1 yellow squash, thinly sliced

For the Herb-Infused Oil
- 1/4 cup olive oil
- 1 garlic clove, minced
- 1 tsp mixed dried herbs (thyme, oregano, rosemary)
- Salt and pepper, to taste

INSTRUCTIONS

1. **Prepare the Crust:** Preheat oven to 375°F (190°C). Mix almond flour, oil, water, and salt to form a dough. Press into a tart pan and prick with a fork. Bake for 15 minutes until lightly golden; cool slightly.

2. **Prepare the Vegetables:** Thinly slice the sweet potato, zucchini, carrot, eggplant, and yellow squash using a mandoline or sharp knife.

3. **Assemble the Tart:** Spread hummus over the crust. Starting from the center, tightly roll a slice of sweet potato into a spiral and place it in the center. Wrap the other vegetable slices around it, alternating colors until the tart edges are reached.

4. **Make Herb-Infused Oil:** Mix olive oil, garlic, herbs, salt, and pepper. Brush over the vegetables for flavor and gloss.

5. **Bake the Tart:** Bake for 40-50 minutes until vegetables are tender and the crust is crispy. Cover with foil if over-browning.

Cooking Method: Baking

NUTRITIONAL INFORMATION (APPROX. PER SERVING)

Calories: 260 kcal | Carbs: 16 g | Fat: 19 g | Fiber: 5 g | Cholesterol: 0 mg | Sodium: 320 mg

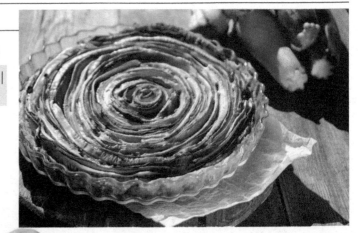

Forest Delight Mushroom Patties

Cooking Time: 40 minutes, Servings: 6 patties

INGREDIENTS

2 cups chopped mushrooms (shiitake or button)

1 medium onion, finely chopped

1 clove garlic, minced

1 cup mashed boiled potatoes

1/2 cup rolled oats

1/4 cup finely chopped fresh dill or parsley

1 tbsp soy sauce

1/2 tsp smoked paprika

Himalayan salt, to taste

1/4 tsp ground cumin

Black pepper, to taste

Olive oil, for frying

INSTRUCTIONS

1. **Prepare the Vegetables:** Heat olive oil in a skillet over medium heat. Add mushrooms, onion, and garlic; sauté until soft and moisture evaporates.

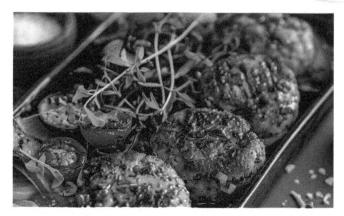

2. **Mix Ingredients:** In a large bowl, combine sautéed mushrooms with mashed potatoes, rolled oats, dill (or parsley), soy sauce, smoked paprika, cumin, salt, and pepper. Mix until uniform.

3. **Form Patties:** Shape the mixture into patties. Add more rolled oats if the mixture is too moist.

4. **Fry Patties:** Heat olive oil in a skillet. Fry patties for 3-4 minutes on each side until golden brown.

NUTRITIONAL INFORMATION (APPROX. PER SERVING)

Calories: 150 kcal | Protein: 5 g | Fat: 5 g | Carbs: 22 g

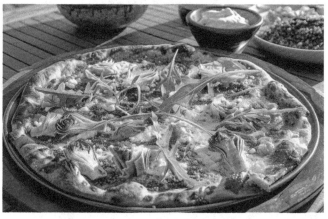

INSTRUCTIONS

1. **Prepare the Crust:** Preheat oven to 350°F (175°C). Mix almond meal, flaxseed mixture, water, baking powder, salt, and olive oil in a bowl to form a sticky dough. Press into a round pizza base (1/4 inch thick) on parchment paper. Transfer to a baking sheet.

2. **Pre-bake the Crust:** Bake for about 15 minutes until golden brown.

3. **Add Toppings:** Spread pesto over the crust. Top with artichoke hearts, sun-dried tomatoes, and dollops of vegan ricotta.

4. **Final Baking:** Return to the oven for 10-15 minutes until heated through and edges are browned.

Pesto Artichoke Pizza with Vegan Ricotta on Almond Meal Crust

Cooking Time: 35 minutes, Servings: 2 (1 medium pizza)

INGREDIENTS

For the Almond Meal Crust

2 cups almond meal

1 tbsp ground flaxseed (mixed with 3 tbsp water; let sit for 5 minutes)

1/4 cup water

1 tsp baking powder

1/2 tsp salt

1 tbsp olive oil

For the Toppings

1/2 cup vegan pesto

1/2 cup artichoke hearts, quartered

1/4 cup sun-dried tomatoes, chopped

1/4 cup vegan ricotta cheese

Fresh basil leaves, for garnish

5. **Garnish and Serve:** Top with fresh basil before slicing and serving.

NUTRITIONAL INFORMATION (APPROX. PER SERVING)

Calories: 650 kcal | Protein: 20 g | Fat: 50 g | Carbs: 30 g | Fiber: 12 g

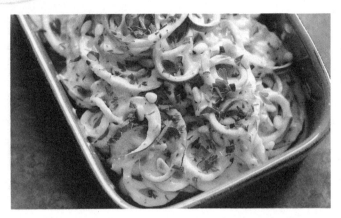

Zucchini Noodle Alfredo

Cooking Time: 20 minutes, Servings: 4

INGREDIENTS

4 large zucchinis, spiralized

1 cup raw cashews, soaked 4+ hours and drained

1/2 cup water

2 tbsp nutritional yeast

1 tbsp lemon juice

2 cloves garlic, minced

1 tbsp Himalayan salt or celery salt

1/2 tsp black pepper

1/4 cup chopped fresh parsley (for garnish)

Optional: Pine nuts for topping

Cooking Method: Blending and boiling.

NUTRITIONAL INFORMATION (APPROX. PER SERVING)

Calories: 250 kcal | Protein: 9 g | Fat: 16 g | Carbs: 18 g

INSTRUCTIONS

1. **Make Sauce:** Blend soaked cashews, water, nutritional yeast, lemon juice, garlic, salt, and pepper until smooth. Adjust seasoning if needed.

2. **Cook Zoodles:** Boil water and blanch zucchini noodles for 1-2 minutes until tender but firm. Drain and keep warm.

3. **Combine:** Toss zucchini noodles with Alfredo sauce in the pot. Serve immediately, garnished with parsley and pine nuts, if desired.

Moroccan Tagine with Apricots and Almonds

Cooking Time: 1 hour, Servings: 4

INGREDIENTS

2 tbsp olive oil (or water/vegetable broth)

1 large onion, chopped

2 cloves garlic, minced

1 tsp ground cumin

1 tsp ground cinnamon

1/2 tsp ground ginger

1/4 tsp ground turmeric

1 can (15 oz) chickpeas, drained and rinsed

1 large carrot, sliced

1 sweet potato, cubed

1 zucchini, sliced

1/2 cup dried apricots, chopped

3 cups vegetable broth

Salt and pepper to taste

1/4 cup toasted almonds, roughly chopped

Fresh cilantro or parsley, for garnish

NUTRITIONAL INFORMATION (APPROX. PER SERVING)

Calories: 350 kcal | Protein: 9 g | Fat: 12 g | Carbs: 55 g

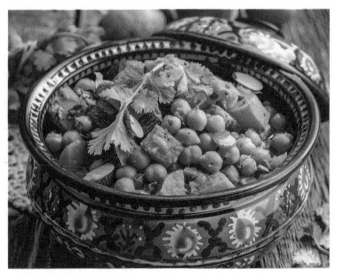

INSTRUCTIONS

1. **Sauté:** In a large pot or tagine, heat oil over medium heat. Sauté onion and garlic until translucent. Add cumin, cinnamon, ginger, and turmeric; cook until fragrant (about 1 minute).

2. **Add Vegetables:** Stir in carrots, sweet potatoes, zucchini, and chickpeas to coat with spices.

3. **Simmer:** Add apricots and vegetable broth. Bring to a boil, then reduce heat to low. Cover and simmer for about 45 minutes until vegetables are tender.

4. **Finish:** Season with salt and pepper. Stir in toasted almonds before serving.

Plant-based Quinoa Paella with Saffron and Artichokes

Cooking Time: 40 minutes, Servings: 4

INGREDIENTS

2 tbsp olive oil (or vegetable broth for oil-free)
1 large onion, finely chopped
2 cloves garlic, minced
1 red bell pepper, sliced
1 green bell pepper, sliced
2 tomatoes, diced
1 cup quinoa, rinsed
1 pinch saffron threads, soaked in 1/4 cup warm water
3 cups vegetable broth
1 cup artichoke hearts, quartered
1/2 cup frozen peas
1/2 cup green olives, sliced
Salt and pepper to taste
Fresh parsley, chopped for garnish
Lemon wedges for serving

NUTRITIONAL INFORMATION (APPROX. PER SERVING)

Calories: 280 kcal | Protein: 9 g | Fat: 7 g | Carbs: 45 g

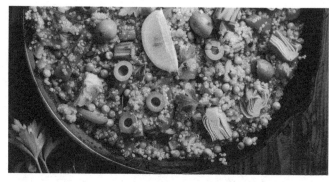

INSTRUCTIONS

1. **Sauté:** In a large skillet or paella pan, heat oil over medium heat. Sauté onion and garlic until translucent. Add bell peppers and cook until softened. Stir in tomatoes and cook until juices are released.

2. **Cook Quinoa:** Add quinoa and mix with vegetables. Pour in saffron-infused water and broth. Bring to a simmer, cover, and cook for about 15 minutes until quinoa is nearly tender.

3. **Add Vegetables:** Stir in artichokes, peas, and olives. Season with salt and pepper. Cook for another 5 minutes until quinoa is fully cooked and liquid is absorbed.

4. **Final Touches:** Remove from heat and let sit for a few minutes for flavors to meld.

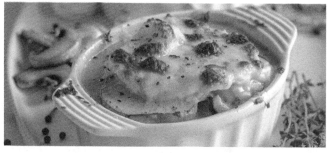

2. **Make Sauce:** Sprinkle mushrooms with cornstarch. Gradually stir in plant-based milk, mixing to prevent lumps. Add nutritional yeast, mustard, salt, pepper, and nutmeg. Cook over low heat for 5-7 minutes until thickened.

3. **Bake:** Preheat oven to 180°C (350°F). Distribute mushroom mixture into baking dishes and top with vegan mozzarella. Bake for 10-15 minutes until golden and melted.

4. **Serve:** Serve hot, garnished with fresh herbs.

Cooking Method: Sautéing and baking.

NUTRITIONAL INFORMATION (APPROX. PER SERVING)

Calories: 200 kcal | Protein: 9 g | Fat: 12 g | Carbs: 17 g | Fiber: 3 g

Mushroom Julien with Plant Based Mozzarella

Prep Time: 30 minutes, Cooking Time: 25-30 minutes, Servings: 4

INGREDIENTS

500 g mushrooms, sliced
1 medium onion, diced
2 cloves garlic, minced
2 tbsp olive oil
1.5 tbsp cornstarch (or arrowroot powder)
1.5 cups plant-based milk (e.g., almond or cashew)
1/4 cup nutritional yeast
1 tsp Dijon mustard
Salt and black pepper to taste
1/4 tsp nutmeg
1 tsp dried thyme or a few sprigs fresh thyme
2 tbsp fresh herbs for garnish (e.g., parsley or dill)
100 g vegan mozzarella, sliced or shredded

INSTRUCTIONS

1. **Sauté Vegetables:** Heat olive oil in a skillet over medium heat. Add onion; cook for 3-4 minutes until translucent. Add garlic and mushrooms; sauté for 5-7 minutes until golden.

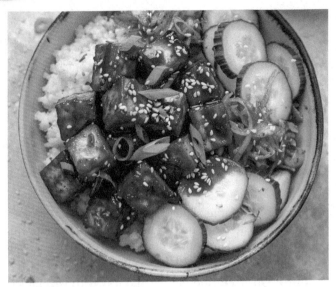

Korean BBQ Tofu Bowls with Cauliflower Rice

Cooking Time: 30 minutes, Servings: 4

INGREDIENTS

1 block (14 oz) firm tofu, pressed and cubed

2 tbsp sesame oil (or water/vegetable broth)

1/4 cup vegan Korean BBQ sauce

1 large head cauliflower, grated into rice-sized pieces

1 small cucumber, thinly sliced

1 carrot, julienned

1/2 cup kimchi

1/4 cup green onions, chopped

1 tbsp sesame seeds

Fresh cilantro, chopped for garnish

INSTRUCTIONS

1. **Make Cauliflower Rice:** Heat a skillet over medium heat. Add sesame oil (or water/broth) and grated cauliflower; sauté for 5-7 minutes until tender. Season lightly with salt and set aside.

2. **Cook Tofu:** In another skillet, heat sesame oil over medium-high heat. Add tofu cubes; fry for 8-10 minutes until golden. Reduce heat, add BBQ sauce, and toss to coat. Cook for an additional 5 minutes.

3. **Assemble Bowls:** Divide cauliflower rice among four bowls. Top with BBQ tofu, cucumber, carrots, and kimchi. Garnish with green onions, sesame seeds, and cilantro.

NUTRITIONAL INFORMATION (APPROX. PER SERVING)

Calories: 250 kcal | Protein: 12 g | Fat: 8 g | Carbs: 18 g

Pearl Barley Mushroom Risotto

Cooking Time: 60 minutes (plus 2 hours for soaking), Servings: 4

INGREDIENTS

1 cup pearl barley, soaked for 2 hours and drained

2 tbsp olive oil (or vegetable broth for no-oil)

1 small onion, finely chopped

2 cloves garlic, minced

3 cups mixed mushrooms (e.g., cremini, portobello, shiitake)

4 cups warm vegetable broth

1 tbsp fresh thyme leaves

Salt and pepper, to taste

Fresh parsley, chopped for garnish

Optional: Truffle oil, 1/2 cup white wine, 1/4 cup grated vegan Parmesan

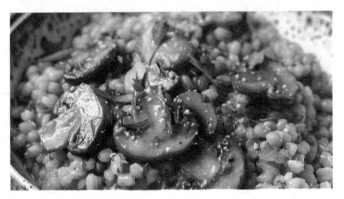

INSTRUCTIONS

1. **Prepare the Barley:** Soak barley for 2 hours, then drain and rinse. In a large pan, heat olive oil over medium heat. Sauté onion and garlic until translucent. Add barley and toast for 2 minutes.

2. **Cook the Mushrooms:** Add mushrooms and cook until juices are released.

3. **Deglaze and Simmer:** If using wine, add it now and reduce by half. Gradually stir in warm broth, one ladle at a time, allowing most liquid to absorb before adding more. Cook until barley is tender, about 45-50 minutes.

4. **Season:** Stir in thyme, salt, pepper, and vegan Parmesan, if using.

NUTRITIONAL INFORMATION (APPROX. PER SERVING)

Calories: 350 kcal | Protein: 8 g | Fat: 10 g | Carbs: 54 g

Roasted Stuffed Bell Peppers with Red Lentils

Cooking Time: 1 hour, Servings: 6

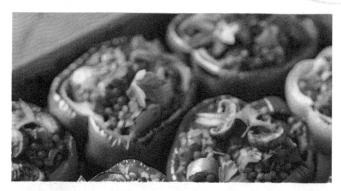

INGREDIENTS

- 6 large bell peppers (any color)
- 1 large carrot, finely chopped
- 1 large onion, finely chopped
- 2 cloves garlic, minced
- 200 g mushrooms, chopped
- 150 g red lentils, pre-cooked
- 1 red bell pepper, finely chopped

- 1 large tomato, diced
- 1 tbsp tomato paste
- 1 tsp dried basil
- 1 tsp dried oregano
- Himalayan salt and black pepper, to taste
- Vegetable broth for sautéing
- Fresh herbs (parsley, basil) for garnish

INSTRUCTIONS

1. **Prepare Peppers:** Preheat oven to 350°F (180°C). Cut tops off peppers, remove seeds, and set aside.
2. **Sauté Vegetables:** In a skillet, heat broth over medium heat. Add carrot, onion, and garlic; sauté for 5 minutes. Add mushrooms and chopped red bell pepper; cook until mushrooms are golden, about 5 minutes.
3. **Add Tomatoes and Seasoning:** Stir in tomatoes, tomato paste, basil, oregano, salt, and pepper. Cover and simmer for 10 minutes.
4. **Add Lentils:** Mix in pre-cooked red lentils.
5. **Stuff Peppers:** Fill each pepper with the vegetable mixture and replace tops. Place in a baking dish.
6. **Bake:** Bake for 30-40 minutes until peppers are tender and slightly browned.

NUTRITIONAL INFORMATION (APPROX. PER SERVING)

Calories: 180 kcal | Protein: 8 g | Fat: 6 g | Carbs: 25 g | Fiber: 7 g

GAS GRILL PARTY: SMOKY AND SPECTACULAR

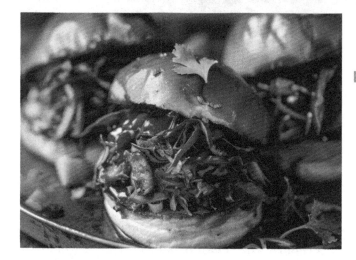

Smoky Barbecue Jackfruit Sliders

Cooking Time: 45 minutes, Servings: 8 sliders

INGREDIENTS:

For the Jackfruit:
- 2 cans young green jackfruit, drained
- 1 onion, sliced
- 2 garlic cloves, minced

For the BBQ Sauce:
- 1 cup tomato sauce
- 1/4 cup apple cider vinegar
- 1/4 cup date puree
- 2 tbsp soy sauce
- 1 tbsp smoked paprika
- 1 tsp mustard powder
- 1 tsp liquid smoke
- Salt, pepper

For the Slaw:
- 2 cups shredded red cabbage
- 1 carrot, shredded
- 1/4 cup apple cider
- vinegar
- 1 tbsp maple syrup
- Salt

INSTRUCTIONS:

1. **Shred jackfruit:** Sauté onion and garlic for 5 minutes.
2. **Mix sauce ingredients:** Add jackfruit, coat with sauce, and simmer for 20-30 minutes.
3. **Combine slaw ingredients:** Toss cabbage and carrot in dressing.
4. **Assemble sliders:** add jackfruit and slaw to buns.

NUTRITIONAL INFORMATION (APPROX. PER SERVING):

Calories: 200 kcal | Protein: 6 g | Fat: 2 g | Carbs: 40 g

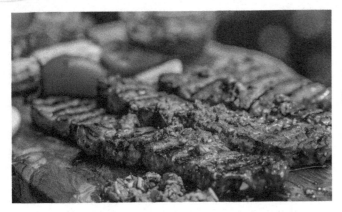

Grilled Seitan Steak with Chimichurri Sauce

Cooking Time: 30 minute, Servings: 4

INGREDIENTS

For the Seitan Steaks:

500	1 tbsp smoked paprika
2 tbsp soy sauce	1 tsp garlic
1 tbsp olive oil	1 tsp onion powder

For the Chimichurri Sauce:

1 cup fresh parsley, finely chopped	1/2 cup olive
1/4 cup	2 tbsp red wine vinegar
3 cloves garlic, minced	1 tsp chili flakes
	Salt and pepper, to t

Cooking Method: Grilling.

NUTRITIONAL INFORMATION (APPROXIMATE PER SERVING)

Calories: 350 k | Protein: 28 g | Fat: 25 g | Carbs: 9 g | Fiber: 2

INSTRUCTIONS

1. **Marinate the Seitan:** In a bowl, mix soy sauce, olive oil, smoked paprika, garlic powder, and onion powder. Coat the seitan steaks evenly and marinate for at least 20 minutes.

2. **Prepare the Chimichurri Sauce:** In a small bowl, combine parsley, oregano, garlic, olive oil, vinegar, chili flakes, salt, and pe

3. **Grill the Seitan Steaks:** Preheat grill to medium-high heat. Grill seitan steaks for about 5 minutes on e

4. **Serve:** Top grilled seitan steaks with chimichurri sauce.

Grilled Tempeh and Vegetable Kebabs with Peanut Sauce

Cooking Time: 25 minutes, Servings: 4

INGREDIENTS

For the Kebabs:

400 g tempeh, cubed	2 medium zucchinis, sliced into rounds
1 red bell pepper, cubed	1 large onion, chunked
1 yellow bell pepper, cubed	

Marinade:

3 tbsp soy sauce	1 tsp ground coriander
2 tbsp olive oil	1 tbsp honey or agave nectar
1 tbsp vinegar	

For the Peanut Sauce:

1/2 cup peanut butter	Warm water (as needed)
2 tbsp soy sauce	Optional: 1/2 tsp chili flakes
1 tbsp lime juice	
2 tsp honey or agave nectar	

NUTRITIONAL INFORMATION (APPROX. PER SERVING)

Calories: 320 kcal | Protein: 19 g | Fat: 18 g | Carbs: 22 g | Fiber: 5 g

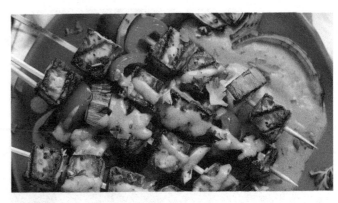

INSTRUCTIONS

1. **Marinate the Ingredients:** In a large bowl, mix soy sauce, olive oil, vinegar, coriander, and honey/agave. Add tempeh, bell peppers, zucchini, and onion, tossing to coat. Marinate for at least 15 minutes.

2. **Prepare the Peanut Sauce:** In a small bowl, combine peanut butter, soy sauce, lime juice, honey/agave, and chili flakes. Gradually add warm water to reach desired consistency.

3. **Assemble the Kebabs:** Thread marinated tempeh and vegetables onto skewers.

4. **Grill the Kebabs:** Preheat grill to medium heat. Grill kebabs for 10-15 minutes, turning occasionally, until vegetables are tender and tempeh is charred.

Cauliflower Steak with Herb Salsa Verde

Cooking Time: 30 minutes, Servings: 4

INGREDIENTS

For the Cauliflower Steaks:

2 large heads of cauliflower

2 tbsp olive oil (or a spray of water for a low-oil version)

Salt and pepper to taste

For the Herb Salsa Verde:

1/2 cup chopped fresh parsley

1/4 cup chopped fresh cilantro

2 tbsp chopped fresh mint

1 clove garlic, minced

Zest and juice of 1 lemon

2 tbsp capers, chopped

1/2 cup olive oil (or less, based on preference)

Salt and pepper to taste

NUTRITIONAL INFORMATION (APPROX. PER SERVING)

Calories: 280 kcal | Protein: 5 g | Fat: 25 g | Carbs: 12 g

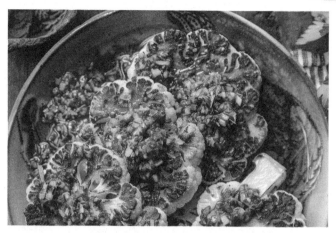

INSTRUCTIONS

1. **Prepare the Cauliflower Steaks:** Preheat oven to 400°F (200°C). Remove cauliflower leaves and trim the stem. Cut each head into 1-inch thick slices, ensuring some core remains. Brush with olive oil or spray with water, then season with salt and pepper. Roast on a baking sheet for 25 minutes, turning once, until golden and tender.

2. **Make the Herb Salsa Verde:** In a bowl, combine parsley, cilantro, mint, garlic, lemon zest, lemon juice, and capers. Slowly whisk in olive oil until blended. Season with salt and pepper.

SIDE DISHES AND SNACKS: PERFECT COMPLEMENTS

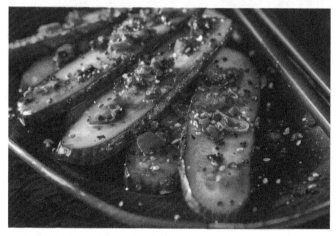

Fiery Eastern Cucumber Fans

Preparation Time: 15 minutes, Servings: 4

INGREDIENTS

2 large cucumbers

1 tbsp sesame oil

2 tbsp soy sauce

1 tbsp rice or apple cider vinegar

2 cloves garlic, minced

1 tsp fresh ginger, grated

1 tsp red chili pepper, minced (or flakes)

1 tbsp date puree (blend dates with water)

2 stalks green onions, chopped

1 tsp sesame seeds

INSTRUCTIONS

1. **Prepare Cucumbers:** Slice cucumbers lengthwise into quarters or halves. If watery, sprinkle with salt, let sit for 10 minutes, then drain excess liquid.

2. **Make the Marinade:** In a bowl, mix sesame oil, soy sauce, vinegar, garlic, ginger, chili, and date puree.

3. **Combine:** Place cucumbers in a deep bowl, pour marinade over, and mix to coat evenly.

NUTRITIONAL INFORMATION (PER SERVING)

Calories: 75 Kcal | Fat: 4.5 g | Carbs: 9 g | Protein: 2 g | Sodium: 570 mg | Fiber: 2 g

Plant-based Based Aspic with Agar-Agar

Cooking Time: 1 hour, Servings: 6

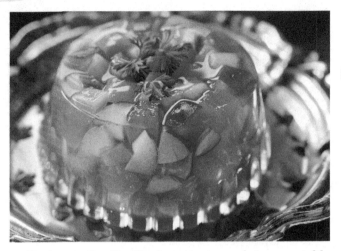

INGREDIENTS

2 cups vegetable broth

2 tsp agar-agar

1 carrot, thinly sliced

1 small parsley root, diced

1 small celery root, diced

100 g green peas (fresh or frozen)

1 red bell pepper, diced

1 small onion, thinly sliced

Juice of 1 lemon

Salt and black pepper, to taste

Fresh dill for garnish

INSTRUCTIONS

1. **Prepare the Vegetables:** Boil carrots, parsley root, and celery in a small amount of water for 5 minutes. Add green peas and cook for 2 more minutes. Drain.

2. **Prepare the Broth:** In a saucepan, bring vegetable broth to a boil, add agar-agar, and simmer for 2 minutes.

3. **Assemble the Aspic:** In a mold, layer the vegetables and pour some agar-agar broth over them. Repeat until the mold is filled, leaving some space for shrinkage.

4. **Setting:** Cool at room temperature, then refrigerate for 3-4 hours until set.

NUTRITIONAL INFORMATION (APPROX. PER SERVING)

Calories: 50 kcal | Protein: 2 g | Fat: 0.5 g | Carbs: 11 g | Fiber: 3 g

---

Baked Vegan Spring Rolls with Rice Paper

Cooking Time: 30 minutes, Servings: 4 (makes about 12 rolls)

INGREDIENTS

For the Spring Rolls:

12 rice paper wrappers

1 cup red cabbage, thinly sliced

1 cup carrots, julienned

1 cup bell peppers, julienned

1 cup cucumber, thinly sliced

1/2 cup fresh mint leaves

1/2 cup fresh basil leaves

1/4 cup green onions, finely chopped

2 tbsp sesame seeds (for garnish)

Olive oil or cooking spray

For the Dipping Sauce:

1/4 cup soy sauce

2 tbsp rice vinegar

1 tbsp sesame oil

Optional: 1 tsp chili sauce or sriracha

1 tsp grated ginger

1 clove garlic, minced

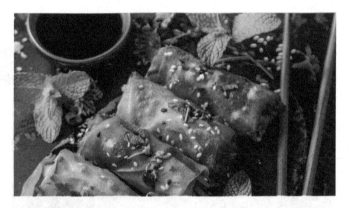

INSTRUCTIONS

1. **Preparation:** Preheat oven to 400°F (200°C) and line a baking sheet with parchment paper.

2. **Hydrate the Rice Paper:** Dip each rice paper wrapper in warm water for 10-15 seconds until soft.

3. **Assemble the Spring Rolls:** Place a small handful of vegetables and herbs on the lower third of the wrapper. Fold the bottom over the filling, tuck in the sides, and roll tightly. Repeat with remaining ingredients.

4. **Bake:** Arrange rolls on the baking sheet, brush tops with olive oil, and bake for 20-25 minutes, turning halfway, until golden and crispy.

5. **Prepare the Dipping Sauce:** Whisk together all sauce ingredients in a bowl, adjusting seasoning as desired.

NUTRITIONAL INFORMATION (APPROXI. PER SERVING)

Calories: 200 kcal | Protein: 4 g | Fat: 5 g | Carbs: 35 g | Fiber: 3 g

Spinach and Green Pea Falafel with Mint Dressing

Cooking Time: 35 minutes, Servings: 4 (about 12 falafels)

INGREDIENTS

For the Falafels:

1 cup raw chickpeas, soaked overnight and drained

1 cup fresh spinach, chopped

1/2 cup green peas (fresh or thawed)

2 cloves garlic, minced

1 small onion, finely chopped

1 tsp ground cumin

1/2 tsp ground coriander

Juice of 1 lemon

1/4 cup fresh mint, chopped

2 tbsp ground flaxseeds

Himalayan salt or celery salt, to taste

For the Mint Dressing:

1/2 cup unsweetened plant-based yogurt

1/4 cup fresh mint, finely chopped

1 tbsp lemon juice

1 clove garlic, minced

Salt, to taste

NUTRITIONAL INFORMATION (APPROX. PER SERVING)

Calories: 200 kcal | Protein: 8 g | Fat: 4 g | Carbs: 33 g | Fiber: 7 g

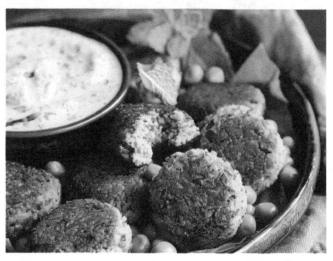

INSTRUCTIONS

1. **Prepare the Falafel Mixture:** Blend chickpeas, spinach, green peas, garlic, onion, cumin, coriander, lemon juice, and mint in a food processor until chunky. Add ground flaxseeds and season with salt.

2. **Shape and Cook:** Form the mixture into balls or patties. Place on a parchment-lined baking sheet and bake at 375°F (190°C) for 20-25 minutes, flipping halfway, until golden and firm.

3. **Make the Mint Dressing:** Mix plant-based yogurt, chopped mint, lemon juice, minced garlic, and salt in a bowl until smooth.

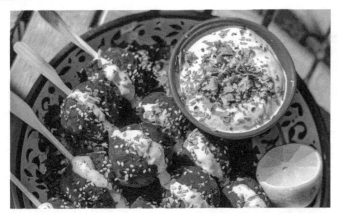

Beetroot Falafel with Tahini-Yogurt Dressing

Cooking Time: 40 minutes, Servings: 4 (about 12 falafels)

INGREDIENTS

For the Falafels:

1 cup raw chickpeas, soaked overnight and drained

1 medium beetroot, peeled and grated

1 small onion, chopped

2 cloves garlic, minced

1 tsp ground cumin

1 tsp ground coriander

1/2 tsp chili powder

1/4 cup fresh parsley, chopped

1/4 cup fresh cilantro, chopped

Juice of 1 lemon

1 tbsp chickpea flour (if needed, for binding)

Himalayan salt, to taste

For the Tahini-Yogurt Dressing:

1/2 cup unsweetened plant-based yogurt

2 tbsp tahini

1 tbsp lemon juice

1 clove garlic, minced

Salt, to taste

INSTRUCTIONS

1. **Prepare the Falafel Mixture:** Blend soaked chickpeas, beetroot, onion, garlic, spices, parsley, cilantro, and lemon juice in a food processor until textured. Add chickpea flour if too wet. Season with salt.

2. **Shape the Falafels:** Form into balls or patties with damp hands.

3. **Bake:** Preheat oven to 375°F (190°C). Place falafels on a parchment-lined baking sheet and bake for 25-30 minutes, flipping halfway, until crispy.

4. **Make the Dressing:** Whisk yogurt, tahini, lemon juice, garlic, and salt in a bowl until smooth.

NUTRITIONAL INFORMATION (APPROX. PER SERVING)

Calories: 230 kcal | Protein: 9 g | Fat: 6 g | Carbs: 36 g | Fiber: 10 g

---

Crispy Baked Kale Chips Recipe

Cooking Time: 20 minutes, Servings: 4

INGREDIENTS

1 large bunch kale, washed and dried

1 tbsp olive oil

2 tbsp nutritional yeast

1/2 tsp garlic powder

1/4 tsp salt

1/8 tsp black pepper

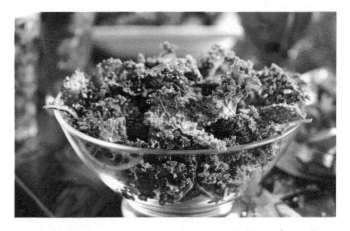

INSTRUCTIONS

1. **Preheat Oven:** Preheat oven to 300°F (150°C). Line a baking sheet with parchment paper. Remove kale leaves from stems and tear into bite-sized pieces.

2. **Season Kale:** In a bowl, drizzle kale with olive oil, then add nutritional yeast, garlic powder, salt, and pepper. Toss to coat evenly.

3. **Bake:** Spread kale in a single layer on the baking sheet. Bake for 10 minutes, flip the leaves, and bake for another 10 minutes until crispy.

4. **Cool and Serve:** Let cool on the baking sheet for a few minutes. Serve immediately or store in an airtight container for up to a week.

NUTRITIONAL INFORMATION (APPROX. PER SERVING)

Calories: 100 kcal | Protein: 3 g | Fat: 5 g | Carbs: 12 g | Fiber: 2

Sweet Potato and Black Bean Quesadillas

Cooking Time: 30 minutes, Servings: 4

INGREDIENTS:

2 large sweet potatoes, peeled and cubed

1 can (15 oz) black beans, rinsed and drained

1 tsp ground cumin

1/2 tsp smoked paprika

Salt and pepper to taste

8 grain-free taco tortillas made with almond and coconut (recipe below) or gluten-free tortillas

1 cup grated plant-based cheese (such as vegan mozzarella or cheddar)

Olive oil or cooking spray for cooking

For the Avocado-Lime Dipping Sauce:

1 ripe avocado

Juice of 1 lime

1 clove garlic, minced

Salt and pepper to taste

Water to thin, as needed

Grain-Free Taco Tortillas with Almond and Coconut:

1 cup almond meal

1/4 cup coconut flour

2 tbsp psyllium husk powder

1/4 tsp sea salt

1 cup hot water (adjust as needed)

Optional: 1/2 tsp cumin or garlic powder for extra flavor

INSTRUCTIONS:

1. **Prepare the Tortillas:** In a large bowl, mix the almond meal, coconut flour, psyllium husk powder, salt, and any optional spices until well combined. Gradually add the hot water, stirring continuously until a dough forms. It should be pliable but not sticky; add more water if it's too dry. Divide the dough into eight equal portions. Roll each portion into a ball. Place a dough ball between two pieces of parchment paper and flatten it with a rolling pin or tortilla press to your desired thickness, about the size of a standard tortilla. Heat a non-stick skillet over medium heat. Cook each tortilla on each side for 1-2 minutes until they are lightly golden and have brown spots. They should be flexible and soft.

2. **Prepare the Sweet Potatoes:** Boil the sweet potatoes in salted water for about 15 minutes until tender. Drain and mash them in a bowl. Season with salt, pepper, cumin, and smoked paprika.

3. **Prepare the Black Beans:**Prepare the Black Beans: Mash the black beans in a separate bowl, keeping some texture. Season with a pinch of salt and pepper.

4. **Make the Avocado-Lime Dipping Sauce:** Combine the avocado, lime juice, minced garlic, salt, and pepper in a blender. Blend until smooth. Add water as necessary to achieve a creamy dipping consistency. Set aside.

5. **Assemble the Quesadillas:** Heat a skillet over medium heat and lightly oil or spray with cooking spray. Spread a layer of mashed sweet potatoes and a spoonful of black beans on one tortilla, generously sprinkle with plant-based cheese, and top with another tortilla. Cook the quesadilla on each side for 3-4 minutes until the tortilla is crispy and the cheese has melted. Repeat with the remaining tortillas and filling.

6. **Serve:** Cut the quesadillas into wedges and serve hot with the avocado-lime dipping sauce.

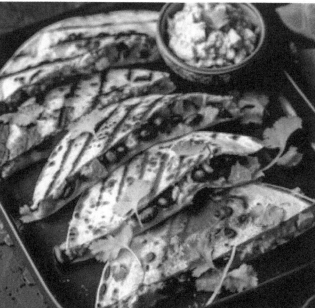

Cooking Method: Frying and boiling.

NUTRITIONAL INFORMATION (APPROX. PER SERVING):

Calories: 350 kcal | Protein: 12 g | Fat: 15 g | Carb: 45 g | Fiber: 8 g

Chapter 6:

SWEETS AND BAKING

BREAD: THE ART OF BAKING

Psyllium Husk Flatbread

Cooking Time: 30 minutes, Serves: 4

INGREDIENTS

- 1 cup oat flour
- 2 tbsp psyllium husk powder
- 1/4 tsp salt
- 1/2 cup warm water
- Optional: spices (cumin, garlic powder, herbs)

Cooking Method: Pan-frying

NUTRITIONAL INFORMATION (APPROX. PER SERVING)

Calories: 120 kcal | Carbs: 18 g | Fat: 2 g | Fiber: 4 g

INSTRUCTIONS

1. **Mix Dry Ingredients:** In a bowl, combine oat flour, psyllium husk powder, salt, and any desired spices.

2. **Create Dough:** Add warm water and mix until a dough forms. Let sit for 5-10 minutes to absorb moisture. Divide into 4 balls and roll out between parchment paper.

3. **Cook:** Heat a non-stick skillet over medium heat. Cook each flatbread for 2-3 minutes on each side until puffed and golden.

4. **Serve:** Enjoy warm.

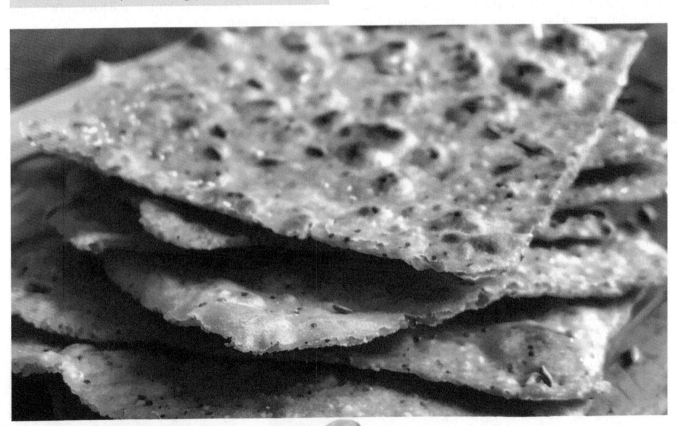

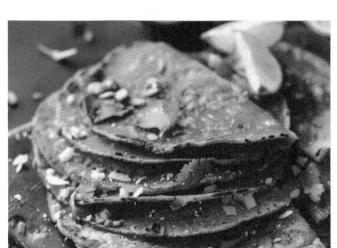

Grain-Free Taco Tortillas with Almond and Coconut

Cooking Time: 20 minutes, Servings: 4 (makes 8 tortillas)

INGREDIENTS

1 cup almond meal
1/4 cup coconut flour
2 tbsp psyllium husk powder
1/4 tsp sea salt

1 cup hot water (adjust as needed)
Optional: 1/2 tsp cumin or garlic powder

INSTRUCTIONS

1. **Mix Dry Ingredients:** In a bowl, combine almond meal, coconut flour, psyllium husk powder, salt, and any optional spices.

2. **Create Dough:** Gradually add hot water, stirring until a pliable, non-sticky dough forms. Add more water if too dry.

3. **Shape Tortillas:** Divide dough into 8 portions, rolling each into a ball. Place a ball between parchment paper and flatten to desired thickness.

4. **Cook:** Heat a non-stick skillet over medium heat. Peel off one side of parchment, flip tortilla into the skillet, then remove the other piece. Cook for 1-2 minutes on each side until lightly golden.

5. **Keep Warm:** Wrap cooked tortillas in a kitchen towel until ready to serve.

Cooking Method: Pan-frying

NUTRITIONAL INFORMATION (APPROX. PER SERVING)

Calories: 150 | Carbs: 8 g | Fat: 10 g | Fiber: 5 g | Cholesterol: 0 mg | Sodium: 150 mg

---

Chickpea Taco Tortillas

Cooking Time: 25 minutes, Servings: 4 (makes eight tortillas)

INGREDIENTS:

1 cup chickpea flour (besan)
1 1/4 cups warm water
1/2 tsp cumin
1/2 tsp paprika
Salt to taste
Olive oil for cooking

INSTRUCTIONS:

1. **Mix Wet and Dry Ingredients:** Whisk together chickpea flour, warm water, cumin, paprika, and salt until smooth. Let the batter sit for a few minutes to thicken slightly.

2. **Cook on Skillet:** Heat a lightly oiled, non-stick skillet over medium heat. Pour some batter into the skillet, tilting to spread into a thin layer. Cook 2-3 minutes on each side until the tortilla is golden and the edges lift. Continue with the remaining batter, adding oil as needed.

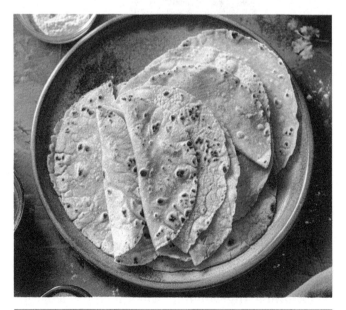

Cooking Method: Pan-frying.

NUTRITIONAL INFORMATION (APPROX. PER SERVING):

Calories: 125 | Carbs: 18 g | Fat: 3 g | Fiber: 3 g | Cholesterol: 0 mg | Sodium: 300 mg

Plant-Based Whole Wheat Bread

Cooking Time: 2 hours 45 minutes (including proofing and baking), Servings: 12 (1 loaf)

INGREDIENTS

2 cups whole wheat flour

1 cup all-purpose flour (or more whole wheat flour)

1 tbsp instant yeast

1 tsp salt

1 tbsp maple or agave syrup

1 and 1/4 cups warm water (approx. 110°F/45°C)

1/4 cup unsweetened applesauce

Optional: 1/2 cup mixed seeds (sunflower, flax, pumpkin, sesame)

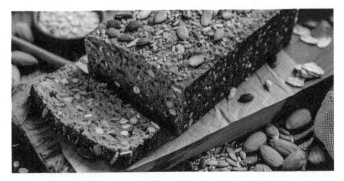

INSTRUCTIONS

1. **Mix Dry Ingredients:** In a large bowl, whisk together whole wheat flour, all-purpose flour, yeast, and salt.

2. **Combine Wet Ingredients:** In a separate bowl, mix warm water and syrup, then add to dry ingredients with applesauce. Stir until a sticky dough forms.

3. **Knead Dough:** Knead on a floured surface for about 10 minutes until smooth and elastic, adding flour as needed.

4. **First Rise:** Place dough in a greased bowl, cover with a damp cloth, and let rise in a warm place for 1 hour or until doubled.

5. **Shape and Second Rise:** Punch down dough, shape into a loaf, and press seeds on top if desired. Cover and let rise for another 30 minutes.

6. **Bake:** Preheat oven to 375°F (190°C). Bake for 35-40 minutes until golden brown and hollow-sounding when tapped.

7. **Cool:** Let cool on a wire rack before slicing.

NUTRITIONAL INFORMATION (APPROX. PER SERVING)

Calories: 140 | Carbs: 29 g | Fat: 1 g | Dietary Fiber: 4 g | Cholesterol: 0 mg | Sodium: 200 mg

---

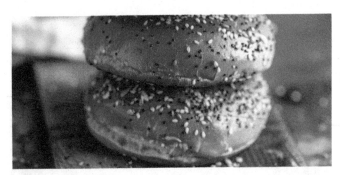

INSTRUCTIONS

1. **Prepare Flax Eggs:** Mix 3 tbsp flaxseed meal with 9 tbsp water. Stir and let sit for 15 minutes until thickened.

2. **Preheat Oven:** Preheat oven to 350°F (175°C) and line a baking sheet with parchment paper.

3. **Mix Dry Ingredients:** In a large bowl, combine almond flour, ground flaxseed, coconut flour, baking powder, and salt.

4. **Combine Ingredients:** Whisk prepared flax eggs, almond milk, and oil in another bowl. Pour into dry ingredients and mix until a sticky dough forms.

5. **Shape Buns:** Divide dough into 4 parts. Shape into buns with moistened hands and place on the baking sheet. Optionally, sprinkle with sesame seeds and press lightly.

Golden Almond Harmony Buns

Cooking Time: 20 minutes, Servings: 4 buns

INGREDIENTS

2 cups almond flour

1/2 cup ground flaxseed (plus 3 tbsp for flax eggs)

1 tbsp coconut flour

1 tsp baking powder

1/2 tsp salt

3 tbsp flaxseed meal (for eggs)

9 tbsp water (for flaxseed)

1/4 cup unsweetened almond milk

2 tbsp olive oil or melted coconut oil

Optional: Sesame seeds for topping

6. **Bake:** Bake for 15-18 minutes until golden brown and a toothpick comes out clean.

7. **Cool and Serve:** Let cool on the baking sheet for a few minutes, then transfer to a wire rack. Slice horizontally once cooled for burgers.

NUTRITIONAL INFORMATION (APPROX. PER SERVING)

Calories: 345 | Protein: 14 g | Fat: 28 g | Carbs: 12 g

DESSERTS: A NEW ERA OF INDULGENCE

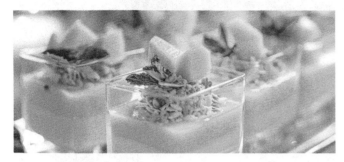

INSTRUCTIONS

1. **Prepare Panna Cotta:** In a saucepan, combine coconut milk, agave syrup, and vanilla. Sprinkle agar-agar over the mixture and let hydrate for 5 minutes. Heat over medium, stirring until boiling, then simmer for 2-3 minutes until dissolved. Pour into glass cups and refrigerate for 1 hour.

2. **Prepare Mango Layer:** Blend chopped mango, lime juice, and agave syrup until smooth. Once the panna cotta sets, carefully pour the mango mixture over it. Chill for another 3 hours until fully set.

3. **Garnish and Serve:** Top each serving with fresh mango slices, mint leaves, and toasted coconut flakes before serving.

Mango and Coconut Panna Cotta with Agave Syrup

Cooking Time: 15 minutes (plus 4 hours chilling), Servings: 4

INGREDIENTS

For the Panna Cotta

400 ml coconut milk	1 tsp vanilla extract
1/4 cup agave syrup	2 tsp agar-agar powder

For the Mango Layer

2 ripe mangoes, peeled and chopped	Juice of 1 lime
	2 tbsp agave syrup

For Garnishing

Fresh mango slices	Toasted coconut flakes
Mint leaves	

Cooking Method: Stovetop for coconut, blending for mango layer.

NUTRITIONAL INFORMATION (APPROX.PER SERVING)

Calories: 250 | Fat: 15 g | Carbs: 28 g | Fiber: 3 g | Sugars: 24 g | Protein: 2 g | Sodium: 15 mg

---

Dessert Pavlova "Berry Cloud"

Cooking Time: 2 hours, Servings: 6-8

INGREDIENTS

For the Meringue

1 cup aquafaba	1 cup coconut sugar (or erythritol for strict plant-based)
1/4 tsp cream of tartar	
1 tsp vanilla extract	

For the Cream

1 can cold coconut milk (solid part only)	3 tbsp maple syrup
	1/2 tsp vanilla extract

For Garnish

Fresh berries (strawberries, raspberries, blueberries, blackberries)

Edible flowers

Mint leaves

Coconut sugar powder (or erythritol powder for strict plant-based)

INSTRUCTIONS

1. **Meringue Preparation:** Preheat the oven to 212°F (100°C) and line a baking sheet with parchment paper. Beat aquafaba with cream of tartar until soft peaks form. Gradually add sugar and whip until glossy, stiff

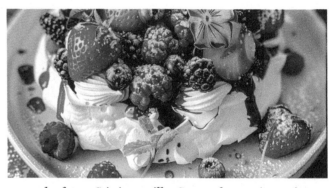

peaks form. Stir in vanilla. Spoon the meringue into a round shape with a well in the center. Bake for 1.5–2 hours until dry and easily peels away. Cool completely in the oven.

2. **Cream Preparation:** Whip the solid coconut milk with maple syrup and vanilla until thick.

3. **Assemble the Dessert:** Spread the cream over the cooled meringue. Top with fresh berries, edible flowers, and mint leaves. Dust lightly with coconut sugar or erythritol before serving.

NUTRITIONAL INFORMATION (APPROX. PER SERVING)

Calories: 250 | Fat: 10 g | Carbohydrates: 35 g (sugar variations may alter this) | Protein: 2 g | Sodium: 20 mg | Fiber: 3 g

Quinoa and Apple Bake

Prep Time: 30 minutes, Cooking Time: 45 minutes, Servings: 6

INGREDIENTS

1 cup quinoa

2 cups water

3 large apples, diced

1 tsp cinnamon

1/4 cup chopped nuts (walnuts or pecans)

1/4 cup raisins or chopped dates

2 tbsp flaxseed (soaked in 6 tbsp water)

Optional: Coconut oil for greasing

1/2 tsp nutmeg

1/4 tsp cloves

1/4 tsp ginger

INSTRUCTIONS

1. **Prepare Quinoa:** Rinse quinoa in cold water. In a saucepan, bring 2 cups water to a boil. Add quinoa, reduce heat to low, cover, and cook for 15 minutes until absorbed. Let cool.

2. **Prepare Fruit Mixture:** In a bowl, mix diced apples with cinnamon, nutmeg, cloves, and ginger.

3. **Assemble:** Preheat oven to 350°F (175°C). Grease a baking dish with coconut oil. Combine cooled quinoa with the apple mixture, nuts, raisins, and soaked flaxseed. Stir and transfer to the dish.

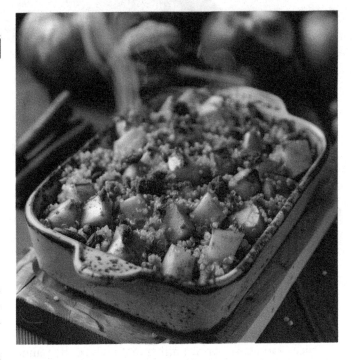

4. **Bake:** Bake for 45 minutes until golden brown.

NUTRITIONAL INFORMATION (APPROX. PER SERVING)

Calories: 220 kcal | Fat: 5 g | Carbs: 38 g | Protein: 6 g | Fiber: 5 g

---

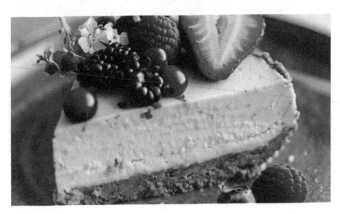

Cashew and Berry Vegan Cheesecake

Cooking Time: 4 hours 30 minutes (including freezing), Servings: 12

INGREDIENTS

For the Crust:

1 cup raw almonds

1 cup pitted dates

1/4 cup melted coconut oil

For the Filling:

2 cups cashews (soaked for 4 hours and drained)

1/2 cup coconut milk

1/2 cup agave syrup

Juice of 1 lemon

1 tsp vanilla extract

1/2 cup berries (fresh or frozen) for garnish

INSTRUCTIONS

1. **Prepare the Crust:** Blend almonds and dates in a blender until crumbly. Add melted coconut oil and blend until moist. Press into the bottom of a cheesecake pan.

2. **Make the Filling:** Blend soaked cashews, coconut milk, agave syrup, lemon juice, and vanilla extract until creamy. Pour over the crust.

3. **Freeze:** Freeze for 4 hours or until firm.

4. **Serve:** Garnish with fresh or frozen berries before serving.

NUTRITIONAL INFORMATION (APPROX. PER SERVING)

Calories: 300 kcal | Carbs: 23 g | Fat: 20 g | Fiber: 3 g | Cholesterol: 0 mg | Sodium: 10 mg

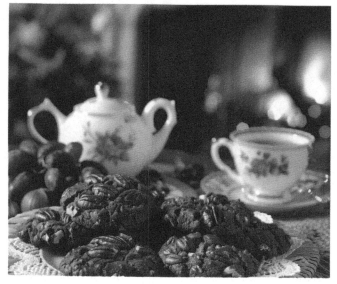

Carob Chip Oatmeal Cookies

Cooking Time: 25 minutes, Servings: 12

INGREDIENTS

1 1/2 cups rolled oats

1 cup almond meal (or finely ground almonds)

1/2 cup carob chips

1/2 cup unsweetened shredded coconut

1/4 cup maple syrup (or agave syrup)

1/4 cup coconut oil (melted)

1/4 cup unsweetened applesauce

1 tsp vanilla extract

1/2 tsp baking soda

1/4 tsp salt

Optional: 1/2 cup chopped walnuts or pecans

INSTRUCTIONS

1. **Preheat:** Oven to 350°F (175°C). Line a baking sheet with parchment paper.

2. **Mix Dry Ingredients:** In a bowl, combine oats, almond meal, carob chips, coconut, and nuts (if using).

3. **Mix Wet Ingredients:** In another bowl, whisk together maple syrup, melted coconut oil, applesauce, and vanilla extract.

4. **Combine:** Add wet ingredients to dry, then sprinkle with baking soda and salt. Stir until combined.

5. **Prepare for Baking:** Scoop tablespoons of dough onto the prepared sheet. Flatten slightly. Bake for 10-12 minutes or until edges are golden.

6. **Cool:** Let cool on the sheet for a few minutes before transferring to a wire rack.

NUTRITIONAL INFORMATION (APPROX. PER SERVING)

Calories: 150-200 kcal (varies with nuts) | Carbs: 15 g | Fat: 10 g | Fiber: 3 g | Cholesterol: 0 mg | Sodium: 75 mg

Bliss Balls (Plant-Based Raffaello)

Cooking Time: 15 minutes, Servings: 12 balls

INGREDIENTS

1 cup unsweetened shredded coconut (plus extra for coating)

1/2 cup raw cashews (soaked for 4 hours and drained)

1/4 cup coconut cream

2 tbsp coconut oil

1 tbsp monk fruit sweetener (or other natural sweetener, to taste)

1 tsp vanilla extract

Whole almonds (for the center of each ball)

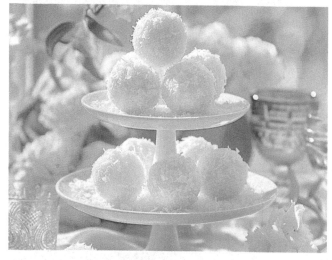

INSTRUCTIONS

1. **Process Ingredients:** In a food processor, blend shredded coconut, soaked cashews, coconut cream, coconut oil, monk fruit sweetener, and vanilla until smooth and holds together.

2. **Form the Balls:** Take a small amount of the mixture, place a whole almond in the center, and roll into a ball. Repeat until the mixture is used.

3. **Coat the Balls:** Roll each ball in extra shredded coconut until well coated.

4. **Chill:** Place balls on a parchment-lined baking sheet and refrigerate for at least an hour or until firm.

NUTRITIONAL INFORMATION (APPROX. PER SERVING)

Calories: 100 kcal | Fat: 9 g | Carbs: 3 g | Protein: 2 g

Florentine Delights

INGREDIENTS

For the Chocolate Base:

1/2 cup raw cocoa powder

1/2 cup melted coconut oil

1/2 cup raw coconut nectar or agave syrup

Pinch of vanilla extract

Pinch of Himalayan salt

For the Topping:

Assorted nuts (almonds, pecans, walnuts), roughly chopped

Dried fruits (raisins, prunes, candied citrus peels, dates), chopped

INSTRUCTIONS

1. **Prepare the Chocolate Sauce:** In a bowl, mix cocoa powder, melted coconut oil, coconut nectar/ agave syrup, vanilla, and salt until well combined. Use immediately or store in an airtight container for up to one week.

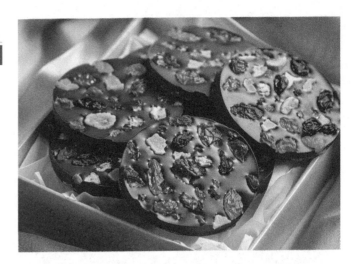

2. **Assemble the Florentines:** In another bowl, combine chopped nuts and dried fruits. Place 1 tablespoon of chocolate sauce into each cup of a silicone or lined muffin tray. Sprinkle with the nut and fruit mixture. Freeze until set.

NUTRITIONAL INFORMATION (APPROX. PER SERVING)

Calories: 200 kcal | Fat: 12 g (varies with nuts) | Carbs: 25 g | Protein: 3 g | Fiber: 2 g

---

ICE CREAM: THE COOL REVOLUTION

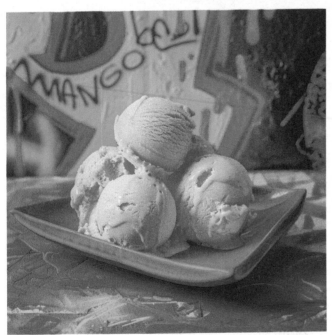

Mango Nice Cream

INGREDIENTS

3 large ripe mangoes, peeled and diced

2 ripe bananas, peeled and sliced

Optional: Juice of 1 lime

INSTRUCTIONS

1. **Prepare the Fruit:** Freeze the mango and banana pieces until solid, ideally overnight. This ensures a creamy texture without added sugars or dairy.

2. **Blend:** In a food processor or blender, combine frozen mango, banana, and lime juice (if using). Blend until smooth and creamy, pausing to scrape down the sides as needed.

3. **Adjust Consistency:** If too thick, add a splash of plant-based milk to facilitate blending, but keep liquid minimal for creaminess.

4. **Serve Immediately:** Enjoy as soft-serve.

5. **Freeze for Later:** For a firmer texture, transfer to an airtight container and freeze for 2-3 hours. Scoop and serve.

NUTRITIONAL INFORMATION
(APPROX. PER SERVING, WITHOUT OPTIONAL INGREDIENTS)

Calories: 200 kcal | Fat: 0.5 g | Carbs: 50 g | Fiber: 5 g | Protein: 2 g

Chocolate Nice Cream

INGREDIENTS

4 ripe bananas, sliced and frozen

2-3 tbsp cacao or carob powder (to taste)

1/2 tsp vanilla extract (optional)

2 tbsp almond milk or any plant-based milk (optional for creaminess)

Optional add-ins: vegan chocolate chips, peanut butter, or cinnamon

INSTRUCTIONS

1. **Prepare Bananas:** Peel and slice bananas. Freeze on a parchment-lined baking sheet for at least 2-3 hours or overnight.

2. **Blend the Base:** In a food processor or high-speed blender, combine frozen bananas, cacao or carob powder, and vanilla extract (if using). Blend until smooth and creamy, scraping down the sides as needed. Add almond milk if the mixture is too thick.

3. **Customize:** Fold in vegan chocolate chips, peanut butter, or cinnamon, blending for a few seconds to incorporate.

4. **Serve:** Enjoy immediately for a soft-serve texture or transfer to an airtight container and freeze for 2 hours for a firmer texture.

NUTRITIONAL INFORMATION (APPROXIMATE PER SERVING, WITHOUT OPTIONAL ADD-INS)

Calories: 110 kcal | Fat: 0.3 g | Carbs: 28 g | Fiber: 3 g | Protein: 1.3 g | Sugar: 15 g

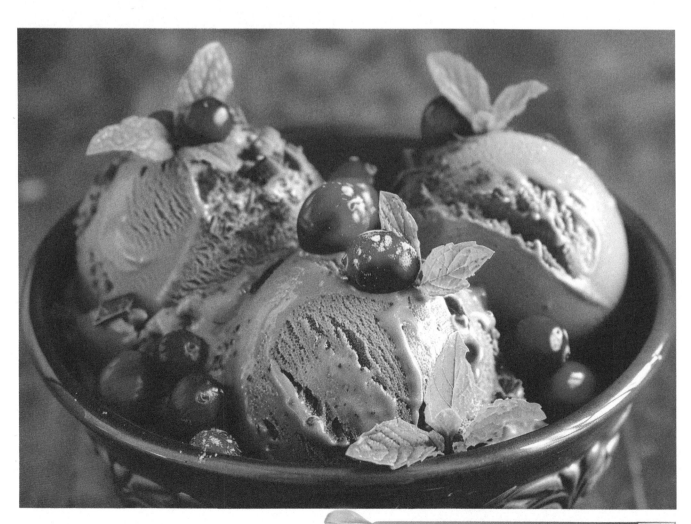

Sugar-Free Almond Vanilla Ice Cream

INGREDIENTS:

2 cups unsweetened almond milk

1 cup soaked cashews (soaked for at least 4 hours and drained)

Seeds from 1 vanilla bean or 1 tbsp pure vanilla extract

1/4 cup xylitol or erythritol (natural sugar alcohols that have a minimal impact on blood sugar)

1/4 tsp guar gum (to improve texture and creaminess)

Optional: 1/4 cup almond butter for added creaminess and flavor

INSTRUCTIONS:

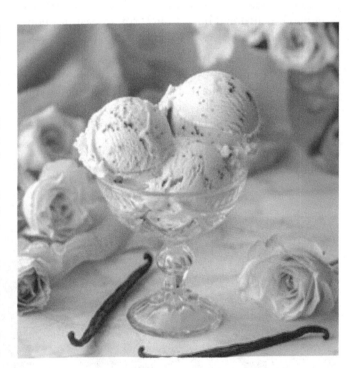

1. **Blend Ingredients:** Combine the almond milk, soaked cashews, vanilla bean seeds (or extract), xylitol or erythritol, and guar gum in a high-speed blender. Blend on high until the mixture is completely smooth. If adding almond butter, include it during this step for extra richness.

2. **Chill the Mixture:** Transfer the mixture to a bowl and refrigerate for at least 2 hours or until well chilled. This step is crucial for achieving the right consistency when churned.

3. **Churn:** Once chilled, pour the mixture into an ice cream maker and churn according to the manufacturer's instructions until it reaches a soft-serve consistency.

4. **Freeze:** Transfer the churned ice cream to an airtight container. Cover the surface with parchment paper to prevent ice crystals, and freeze for at least 4 hours, or until firm.

5. **Serve:** Allow the ice cream to sit at room temperature for 10-15 minutes before serving to soften slightly, making scooping easier.

Cooking Method: Freezing.

NUTRITIONAL INFORMATION (APPROX. PER SERVING):

Calories: 220 kcal | Fat: 18g | Carbs: 8g | Protein: 5g

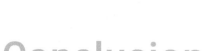

Conclusion

Your Plant-Based Journey Awaits!

Congratulations! You've just taken a significant step towards embracing a healthier, more sustainable, and compassionate way of life. By turning the pages of this cookbook, you've enriched your culinary repertoire and joined a global movement reshaping our relationship with food.

As you've flipped through these recipes, you've seen that plant-based cooking is akin to an artist playing with colors—except your palette is your plate, and your colors are the fresh, vibrant produce that nature provides. And yes, just like any great art, sometimes things might not turn out as expected. Embrace these moments. Laugh at them. Learn from them. And then, eat them anyway—because every masterpiece starts with a brave experiment.

Your journey might have started as a curiosity—can I live happily on a plant-based diet? Hopefully, it's moved toward a resounding "Yes!"—with many more delicious exclamation points along the way. Each recipe you've tried has added to your story, each success has built your confidence, and each mishap... well, it's added to your dinner party anecdotes!

Looking forward, there's a whole community out there, both online and perhaps in your neighborhood, that's also eager to explore plant-based living. You're now a part of this community. Share your experiences, swap recipes, and convert the curious with your now-perfected eggplant parmigiana.

And here's where I leave you, armed with spatulas and inspired by vegetables. I hope this book has been more than just a collection of recipes for you—it's been a companion in your kitchen, a spark for your creativity, and maybe even a mirror reflecting your growth into a savvy, plant-based cook.

So, what's the next step? Continue cooking, continue exploring, and continue sharing your culinary creations. And if you've enjoyed your journey so far, why not spread the word?

If you could take a moment to share your thoughts with a review on Amazon, it would be greatly appreciated—it would also help inspire more people to embark on their plant-based adventures.

Thank you for diving into this journey with my book! Together, let's keep savoring the joy of plant-based cooking and continue to inspire others. Here's to many more delicious discoveries in your kitchen!

Appendix:
Measurement Conversion Tables

This appendix provides detailed conversion tables for measurements commonly used in cooking, which is essential for accurately following recipes, especially in an international context. This section will help readers convert between different units of measurement, making cooking a more accessible and precise activity.

Volume Conversions

This table will help convert liquid volumes between U.S. customary units and metric units.

Volume	US Customary	Metric
1 teaspoon	1tsp	5 milliliters
1 tablespoon	1tbsp	15 milliliters
1 fluid ounce	1 fl oz	30 milliliters
1 cup	1 cup	240milliliters
1 pint	1 pt	473 milliliters
1 quart	1 qt	946 milliliters
1 gallon	1 gal	3.785 liters

Weight Conversions

This table is crucial for converting weights from U.S. customary units to metric units, particularly for dry ingredients.

Weight	US Customary	Metric
1 ounce	1 oz	28.35 grams
1 pound	1 lb	453.59 grams
1/4 pound	4 oz	113.4 grams
1/2 pound	8 oz	226.8 grams
1 kilogram	2.2 lbs	1000 grams

Temperature Conversions

Temperature conversions are critical for cooking, especially when using recipes from countries that use Celsius instead of Fahrenheit.

Temperature	Fahrenheit	Celsius
Oven Low	200°F	93°C
Oven Medium	350°F	177°C
Oven High	400°F	204°C
Water Boils	212°F	100°C
Water Freezes	32°F	0°C

Length Conversions

Occasionally, recipes call for specific cooking dimensions, like the cuts' thickness.

Length	US Customary	Metric
1 inch	1 in	2.54 centimeters
1 foot	12 in	30.48 centimeters

These conversion tables serve as a comprehensive guide for accurately scaling recipes up or down and adapting recipes across different measurement systems, ensuring that anyone can quickly and precisely follow the recipes.

Made in the USA
Coppell, TX
20 February 2025

46195822R00044